Will, My Son

Sarah Boston

Will, My Son
The Life and Death of a Mongol Child

First published in Great Britain by Pluto Press Limited,
Unit 10 Spencer Court, 7 Chalcot Road, London NW1 8LH

Copyright © Sarah Boston 1981

ISBN 0 86104 346 4

Cover designed by Clive Challis
Photoset and printed in Great Britain by
Photobooks (Bristol) Limited, 28 Midland Road, St Philips,
Bristol

Contents

1. Birth / 1
2. The First Ten Days / 9
3. The Tenth Day / 14
4. Limbo Land / 22
5. At Home / 32
6. Settling Down / 46
7. The Future / 54
8. The Choice / 69
9. Death / 81
10. Grief / 87
11. Hiding the Wound / 96
12. A New Life / 102
    How To Find Out More / 113

He weighed 4lbs 6ozs at birth and 14lbs 6ozs at death. He spent 34 weeks in the womb and should have stayed there 40 weeks. He lived for 40 weeks. He should have had 46 chromosomes in each cell but he had 47. He was born on 14 February, St Valentine's Day and died on 20 November. His heart failed him. He was called Will. He was my son.

The bald facts of the brief life of a mentally handicapped child with a severe congenital heart defect might sound to some like a tragic aberration in the normal cycle of human reproduction. As such they regard it as best ended and hopefully forgotten. To me the nine months of his life was an affirmation of life. As such it could never be "best ended" and should not be forgotten.

1. BIRTH

At 8.40 p.m. on 14 February 1975 I gave birth to my first child, a boy weighing 4lbs 6ozs. For me the actual birth was neither a supreme moment of fulfilment, as it is for some women, nor was it the tearing, searing agony that I feared it might be. It was, in some respects, a bit like making love for the first time, a rather bungled affair. By the time I reached the hospital I was well advanced in my labour. The fact that I did not go there earlier was due to two inhibitions. The first was a determined belief, which I clung to even after I had arrived at the hospital, that at six weeks before my expected date of delivery I could not possibly be in labour. The second inhibition was a long conditioned attitude that one shouldn't make a fuss unless one has a serious need to and I wasn't sure that I had such a need. So despite a terrible backache and regular contractions, despite having the classic signs of the onset of labour including a "show" – a small discharge of blood – I drove off across London to have a working lunch with a friend at London Weekend Television.

It was only on my way home, when I stopped to buy some food for our supper, that I realised something distinctly odd was happening to me. At home, after having made myself a cup of tea, I phoned the hospital and as soon as I described my symptoms they advised me to "come in straight away". This instruction I obeyed, helped by two friends who took me there by car. Before they arrived to pick me up I tried to contact Ed, the father of the baby struggling to get out of me, but since he was not in the office I could only leave a message and hope that he would be contacted. At home I left on the kitchen table another note for him and a Valentine present – a plant with heart-shaped leaves.

The time between my arrival at the hospital and the birth of my child passed very quickly. Throughout there seemed to be an endless stream of nurses, midwives and doctors wandering in and out. I tried to implement the breathing patterns that I had learnt in classes run by the National Childbirth Trust but somehow I never got into the rhythm. Partly that was because by that stage I had only done half the course and partly it was because I was not wholly convinced about the power of mind over body. A good "holler", I thought, might be just as good a way of getting through a painful contraction as being very controlled and breathing through it thinking of green pastures or making a cake. I pursued none of these approaches wholeheartedly and breathed a bit, "hollered" a bit, had a bit of pethidine and muddled through.

The one thing that did help me through my labour was the arrival of Ed. One of my friends had stayed with me after I arrived at the hospital and it was reassuring to have her there, but as Ed entered the room I burst into tears. I was so relieved to see him. From the outset of my pregnancy the one thing I had felt sure about was the importance of his presence at the birth of our child. I had felt sure that it would be of critical importance both to "us" and to his relationship with our child. Later his involvement with our child from the moment of birth was to prove to be even more important than I could possibly have imagined.

The second stage of labour was delayed. It soon emerged that I was a bad pusher even though I felt I might burst my bowels with pushing. Ed sat beside me mopping my brow, giving me tiny sips of water and lots of encouragement but none of it helped the baby to come out. Then the doctor decided to intervene. My legs were strung up, I was given an episiotomy (the cutting of the perineum) and my baby was delivered by forceps. The doctor did explain that these measures were necessary since they wanted to get the baby out quickly with the minimum of pressure on its skull, as premature babies have softer, more vulnerable skulls. However, the method of delivery was, I think, one of the main reasons for my feeling that the actual birth was a rather bungled affair.

Then suddenly there it was, my baby, a boy. He cried briefly and it was a wonderful sound. That cry immediately dispelled one of the things I had feared most – a still birth. Quickly he was wrapped up and a nurse was about to rush him out of the room when I said pathetically "can I see my baby?" I was given one quick close look and then he was rushed off. Later I learnt that he had been taken to the premature unit where he could be under intensive care but I don't remember anyone explaining that to me at the time. During my pregnancy I had read nothing about the problems of premature babies so I did not even have any store of information to allay some of my bewilderment.

I was left in the delivery room with my legs still strapped up until the after-birth had been delivered and I had been stitched up. The stitching up was the most painful thing I remember about the whole labour and in retrospect I can't think why, seeing my obvious discomfort, the doctors didn't boost the local anaesthetic.

Cleaned up and changed into a hospital nightdress (I had none of my own) I was wheeled up to the maternity floor. It was then that I resented being in hospital and not at home. More than anything I wanted to be with Ed. We had just had our baby together and it would have been nice to have had a celebratory drink and cuddle together – but no such indulgence was allowed on the hospital ward. Instead we had to kiss each other a demure "goodnight". The next day I found out that after I had been taken up to the ward the doctor took Ed to the intensive care unit and showed him our baby boy already established in his incubator. The doctor also explained to Ed why it was necessary for our baby to be there.

By the time I reached the ward it was after "lights out". I was pleased since I was tired and happy, apart from the absence of Ed, to be left alone. Despite the discomfort of my stitches, allayed by an ice pack, and my worries about my baby which I had barely seen let alone held, I soon fell asleep.

For some women the date of the birth of their first child is one of the most memorable days in their lives. Memorable it certainly was for me but memorable not so much for the particular experiences of the day but as the day when a whole particular, totally unpredicted set of experiences began. I had expected that having a child would inexorably alter the course of my life. I was right. It did change both me and my life. However, my expectations of how it would change were utterly wrong.

For any woman it is almost impossible to know before having a first child how it will affect them and their lives. One can only predict and I predicted the worst.

Looking back I cannot now understand why I got pregnant – or rather why I chose to get pregnant, for it was a conscious choice. The aspects of my life which could be seen as the positive influences were related mainly to the fact that I had established a good strong relationship with Ed, strong and equal. We both worked, shared financial responsibilities, domestic responsibilities (not entirely equally) and both expected to share, in every sense, a child. Ed was more sure that he wanted a child than I was, probably because he could be sure that having a child would alter his life less than mine. However he never pressurised me into making a decision one way or another, realising that the burden of bearing, giving birth and suckling a baby would be mine.

The negative influences seemed much stronger on the surface. They were rooted in my late adolescence and were to do with rational and irrational fears about how a child would affect me and my life.

Up to the time I decided to get pregnant, at the age of thirty, my life had been geared to a "career" or rather to carving out a way of life that enabled me to do the work I enjoyed and be solvent. I had had a privileged middle class upbringing which had not only given me a socially and economically stable childhood but also a lot of encouragement in pursuing academic qualifications in particular. I was supported by my parents at university, applauded by them for getting a reasonably good degree and backed in doing an MA. After leaving university I stumbled into television as a researcher. Quite quickly I realised that my interests in TV lay in documentary film making and so I chose (or rather was pushed into) pursuing that as a freelancer. I realised that to survive I had to diversify my activities and so pursued my other main interest, that of writing. With some ups and considerably more downs I slowly established a satisfying if not very remunerative working life of writing and film making.

Once I knew that I was pregnant and knowing that it would be important for me to keep part of my working life going after having a baby, I set about organising work to make sure that it did. I had been commissioned to write a history book and so I planned to do most of the research work before the birth to enable me to write at home whilst, hopefully, "the baby slept".

Despite my forward planning I still feared the worst. I not only feared that having a baby would at best interrupt and at worst end all that I had worked towards, I also feared the many other ways it might affect my life. When I was about five months pregnant I wrote the following in a diary which rather dramatically sums up what my fears were: "Everything I value will come to an abrupt halt in that tearing, searing, bloody moment of birth. I will no longer be a free agent. Another person's life will be utterly dependent on me. It will take my flesh, my blood, my life and there is no escape. My job opportunities will be severely restricted, my privacy invaded, my time taken and my youth. I fear the effect it will have on my relationship with Ed. I fear the effect it will have on me. I fear for the child I have conceived, my ego trip, whose life is already being moulded inside me."

My equivocal feelings about having a child, feelings which never took into account anything positive *I* would gain from having a child, increased the difficulty I had in coming to terms with being pregnant. One way of trying to evade it was by keeping it a secret from all but Ed and the doctors until I was five months pregnant and the secret could no longer be kept. I did not enjoy being pregnant; I positively hated it. I hated the endless changing physical discomforts. I found it psychologically very hard to re-adjust to both me and my body being taken over by its biological female function. I found it even harder, once it became public, to adjust to, let alone accept, other people's reactions to my pregnant state. I never did come to terms with it but I did, at about six months, mentally and physically reach a kind of stoical commitment to face up to, and try and make the best of, what I felt to be the rather bad situation I had freely chosen to put myself in.

The one decision I did make in late pregnancy which was to be both of short term and, quite unexpectedly, of long term importance to me was my decision to transfer hospitals.

Initially I was registered with a local hospital for the

birth. After attending it once in early pregnancy I took a strong dislike to it. However for most of my pregnancy I forgot about the hospital as I attended the local ante-natal clinic where I was always seen by the same Indian woman doctor. At each visit she was always gentle, patient and personal, hinting from time to time that she knew only too well what it was like being pregnant and to have children of her own. At seven months I reluctantly returned to the hospital clinic and found it as alienating and unsympathetic as on my first visit. I decided to transfer. Not knowing quite how to go about it I phoned up my health visitor who only a day or two previously had informed me that I and my baby-to-be were on her list. I explained my feelings and my wish to be transferred. I also told her where I wished to be transferred to, having done a quick bit of homework on the local hospitals, their attitudes towards childbirth and my friends' experiences of them. To my amazement she said she would see what she could do, commenting that although it was "not the done thing" to transfer and particularly not at this stage of pregnancy, obviously my feelings were all-important. Even more amazing than her attitude was her speedy action. The following day she phoned to say that the transfer had been arranged and that the following week I was to attend St A's where my forms would be.

It was a great relief, the relief being confirmed by my first visit to St A's. There were no hours of unnecessary waiting and the general behaviour of the sister and doctor was quite different from the contemptuous patronising treatment I had received at the first hospital. The feeling that one was on a pregnant production line, whilst not absent, was at least minimised by generally more considerate treatment. The obstetrician I saw was naturally curious about why I had transferred. Although I tried to explain my reasons tactfully, knowing the medical profession tend to close ranks in a defensive stance when any member is criticised, he obviously realised that I had views on how I expected to be treated and responded accordingly.

Later, looking back on the difference between the two hospitals, I realised that it could not be explained entirely by the different personalities and attitudes of the people running the two ante-natal clinics. The difference seemed to lie as much in the class of expectant mother attending each clinic. People tend to be treated as they demand and expect to be treated. The first hospital I attended served an almost entirely working class area of London. It was clear that the women attending the ante-natal clinic neither expected nor demanded any better or more considerate treatment than they got, having been conditioned to accept what was meted out to them by those they saw in authority. In contrast, St A's had attracted a fairly high percentage of middle class expectant mothers, who not only expected and demanded more considerate treatment, but who also, like myself, had the confidence to articulate their expectations. As with education perhaps, the "bussing" of pregnant women would break the ghettos and improve the service but there should be less drastic ways of making all maternity units more considerate.

My transfer was a matter of voting with my feet. At seven months pregnant I was concerned only with my own immediate future – having my baby in a hospital where the attitudes towards childbirth were reasonably progressive and where I felt I was being treated, more or less, as a thinking adult human being. I did not know at that first visit just how immediate the "immediate future" was to be. Much to my surprise and to everyone else's, just over a week after that first visit to St A's my baby was born.

2. THE FIRST TEN DAYS

When I woke up the morning after the birth, or rather when I was woken up, I desperately wanted to see my baby. The feeling was compounded by the fact that all the other mothers in the ward had their babies with them and they were feeding, changing and soothing them. It was not until sometime after breakfast and quite a lot of agitation on my part that finally the sister asked a nurse to accompany me to the premature baby unit. That first visit to the unit was awe-inspiring. Tiny babies in their incubators are even more intimidating to a new mother than a normal sized new-born baby. Having been washed and gowned, I was led over to an incubator and shown my baby. By premature baby standards he wasn't that small but he seemed tiny to me. On that day he was being cared for by a black haired, blue eyed Irish nurse who talked continuously to him in his incubator and included me in the conversation the moment I arrived. Considering he had had a forceps delivery his head appeared relatively unmarked. In fact in general he looked a small but perfectly formed baby with no obvious defects. With no hesitation the nurse disengaged him from the various wires and tubes which were fixed to him; and still talking all the time to him and to me she placed him in my arms to hold.

That was the moment motherhood began for me. I was overwhelmed with all the classic emotions associated with "the maternal instinct"; feelings of tenderness and love, a sense of mystery and bewilderment that I could have produced this tiny, and as I thought, perfect creature. That first time I did not put him to the breast but merely held him. It was enough to create a bond. I wondered at it all. When I returned to the ward I wondered even more at my own reaction. It had taken me completely unawares. I had not expected to be swept off my feet by my own baby.

Fortunately the premature baby unit at St A's was run at that time in a relaxed and humane way, with none of the autocracy and bureaucracy which exists in so many hospitals. The sister in charge did not try to enforce the type of discipline which might have given her a sense of power but which would also have made the development of the relationship between parent and premature baby extremely difficult. On the contrary, considerable lengths were gone to to try and ensure that the parents did establish a relationship with their baby. Ed and I could visit our baby at any time of day or night. Ed normally came to the hospital in the evenings after work and we would visit the unit together. I went on my own several times each day. The nurses were always welcoming and whilst our baby was in the incubator we were never made to feel that it was "a trouble" to any of the nurses to un-tube him and allow us to take him out to hold him. But although the unit was very relaxed I always resented the lack of privacy. I felt inhibited and longed to be able to be on my own with him.

Besides seeing our baby each evening, Ed and I spent a large part of the evening visiting hours trying to think of a name. We had short lists, fads and phases and finally settled on Will. We actually registered him as William Boston Buscombe but he was always called Will.

Those first ten days of Will's life were, in terms of my relationship with him, taken up with the struggle to feed him. In the incubator he was fed by a tube going directly into his stomach. But since I had expressed a desire to breast feed him it was felt he should be put to the breast from the beginning to try to encourage him to suck. Long before his birth I had decided that I wanted to breast feed my baby. For some curious reason the only "romantic" image I had ever held of motherhood was that of the baby at the breast. I was also convinced by other arguments, arguments that the breast *is* best for baby and mother both physically and emotionally.

At my second visit to Will on his first day I started the long struggle to feed him. With the help of the nurse he was gently "put to the breast". He registered no interest. He did not suck, lick, chew, touch or cry. In fact he appeared too sleepy to be interested in anything. His reaction was the same for the next few days. At every feed, or rather attempted feed, I had a nurse with me and in the evening Ed would be there trying to encourage us. With one or two exceptions the nurses were gentle and patient in their help. It was often confusing as different nurses had different theories on the best way to breast feed, but since their advice was usually given sympathetically and not dictatorially I did not feel unduly pressurised to try one way or another. Meanwhile I had to express my milk to keep my production going. What I produced was given to Will.

Expressing milk is a thankless task. It is literally like being a cow and milking oneself. At first I did it with a hand breast pump, then the sister produced a mechanical pump, but finally I found doing it by hand into a sterile jug the most comfortable and dignified way. The only thing that made the whole milk expressing business at that stage bearable was that there were two other mothers, both with babies that couldn't suck, in the premature baby unit, expressing milk too. We chatted, laughed, and joked about "milking time". We had a rota for the mechanical breast pump and had a milk sharing scheme, as one mother produced more milk than her baby needed and I didn't produce enough.

When Will was moved out of his incubator after the first few days into a cot he was changed to a different feeding method. The senior registrar instructed that he was to be spoon-fed. It was explained to me that since I wanted to breast feed him they did not want to put him on a bottle as that would probably make him lazy and mean he would never accept the breast. I gratefully accepted the explanation and continued to try breast feeding him. He continued to show no sign of any sucking reflex. He continued sleepy and unresponsive. He never cried.

At that point I did not question whether Will was any different from any of the other premature babies. It was a common factor that they were sleepy, didn't cry and many did not suck or barely sucked. Will had also had mild jaundice after birth which compounded the sleepiness problem. In contrast, however, to the babies born at term who were with their mothers on the main ward Will seemed tiny, unresponsive and still in the big sleep of the womb.

After about a week odd suspicions did begin to enter my mind. The other premature babies appeared to know *how* to suck but were too lazy or sleepy to bother. I also began to wonder why he was the only one to be spoon-fed when other mothers were equally struggling to teach their babies to breast feed and their babies had been changed from the tube to a bottle. In pursuing that line of unease there seemed nothing concrete for me to grasp. I merely accepted the explanation at face value and thought that Will was obviously just a bit sleepier and slower than the others. Other incidents made me more suspicious. When I asked the obstetrician if it would be possible for me to stay in the hospital for more than my regulation eight days to enable me to be close to Will, he agreed to my request with an almost unnatural enthusiasm. The hospital was generally considerate about allowing mothers to stay, enabling them to be close to their babies who needed to remain in intensive care, so I countered my suspicions by believing that the hospital was just encouraging a close relationship between mother and premature baby. More tangibly worrying was the paediatrician, who said that they "were worried about Will and that they were doing some tests". The results of the tests, he said, would be through by the Monday and he too encouraged me to stay in the hospital, at least until then. I stayed for the weekend and nothing changed. Life was a daily round of hospital routine, punctuated by welcome visits from friends and relatives and the special evening visits of Ed.

What was strange was that despite Will's unresponsive behaviour, both Ed and I felt from the outset that he was a distinctive personality. We felt he was quite definitely a separate, unique human being with his own ways and whims, mainly expressed in his bizarre, wrinkled facial expressions. I had always lumped all new born babies into one categorgy, "babies", and had never realised that a new born child could be so distinctive. Will had immediately established himself as a separate person who was "our baby" and to whom we felt a particular relationship.

3. THE TENTH DAY

It was Monday afternoon during visiting hours that my visitors were interrupted by the appearance of the paediatrician at the doorway to the ward. There were only two mothers in the ward at the time and I assumed that it was me whom he wished to talk to. He hovered in the doorway so I walked across to him. He said that he would like a few words with me and would I mind asking my visitors if they could possibly withdraw so that we could talk in private. I told my parents, who were my visitors, that the paediatrician wished to talk to me on my own and they withdrew somewhere outside the ward.

The sister, the consultant paediatrician, and his junior registrar came over to my bed. The sister pulled the curtains round my bed. I knew then that whatever they were going to say to me was going to be serious. I sat on the edge of my bed, the consultant on a chair almost immediately opposite me, the registrar sat to my right and the sister stood further to my right and outside of my easy vision. The consultant started talking. I remember little of his precise words except that somewhere in those words was the fact that my child was a mongol. "You had been uneasy, you had suspected that something was wrong, hadn't you?" he said, almost appealing to me, as if the fact that I had already suspected that something was wrong would soften the blow. I admitted that I had, but I had never suspected that something was so fundamentally and completely wrong with Will. I started to cry before he had even told me exactly what it was and I continued crying.

At the time I knew nothing about mongolism or mongol babies. I realised it meant handicap, mental retardation, subnormality. An image flashed before my mind of a child with an abnormally large head, the slanted eyes associated with mongolism and a vacant face. That was my image of mongolism culled, I'm not sure from where, but largely from ignorance. The consultant didn't elaborate then on exactly what mongolism was or what caused it. He said only that a test had confirmed it.

I didn't at that stage ask many questions. I was too dazed even to think of any, but I did ask "What will happen to him when he grows up?" Sitting there on the bed a few minutes after having been told that Will was a mongol I somehow thought that I could cope with the prospect of his childhood but what then? The consultant muttered something about sheltered workshops and things being better than they were. I didn't really listen to him. I just saw the rest of my life mapped out – a life inextricably linked to my handicapped child.

The consultant was obviously finding the task of telling me about Will a difficult one, although he must have had considerable experience. The junior registrar was even more uncomfortable. I could see him sitting there hardly daring to look at me and evading my eyes whenever I looked at him. In fact he was a kind, gentle man but both he and his consultant were obviously unschooled in handling such situations.

I was asked again if there were any other questions I wanted to ask. I replied that I was sure there would be but for the moment I couldn't think. I was just stunned. The consultant then asked if I would like him to tell my visitors and I said I would and explained to him that they were my parents. All three then left me. I leant my head on my hands and sobbed.

The next thing I remember was my parents coming in and immediately taking me in their arms and holding me. They too were visibly stunned and upset. My father went to phone Ed. He returned to the ward saying that Ed was out of the office but that he had left a message asking for him to phone the hospital immediately. We sat in the ward and I remember little of what was said.

It was not long before a nurse came to say that Ed was on the phone for me and I could take the call in the sister's office. I went to the office, picked up the phone and stuttered to him, "Please come quickly, just please come quickly to the hospital". He kept saying "What's wrong, what's wrong?" and from the tone of his voice I knew he thought Will was dead. I then just blurted out "He's a mongol". Ed said he was coming and I put the phone down. It was a terrible way to have to break the news to him but I didn't want him to think that Will was dead and there seemed no other way of saying what was wrong. Also I was in the sister's office and knowing that I was being overheard by her and another nurse made me even more uncomfortable. I retreated quickly to my little corner of the ward.

I've never really found out what went through Ed's mind in the taxi between Soho, where he works, and the hospital in West London. But I do know of my relief when he walked in the door of that ward. I saw him, jumped up from my bed, and we just put our arms around each other as we met. We held each other very tight. He then asked me to tell him what the consultant had said about Will. I could answer very few of Ed's questions as I had asked so few questions myself. Ed decided to find the consultant and talk to him, but when Ed returned he seemed to have found out little more than me.

I decided that I would like to go home and be with Ed.

The thought of remaining in hospital separate from him was terrible. The hospital readily agreed that I should be discharged and delegated to my parents the role of keeping a watchful eye on us. They went on ahead of us to open up our house and make it ready for our return. We had one or two things to do before leaving the hospital.

Firstly I had to see a doctor who would discharge me. From the medical point of view this was simple. They were, however, obviously worried about my emotional state and I was prescribed some valium. Having made the decision for me to leave the hospital we decided that we wanted to talk yet again to the consultant paediatrician, but this time together. Mainly we talked about the immediate future. The consultant saw no reason why I shouldn't continue to try to breast feed Will, particularly since we lived fairly near the hospital and could visit regularly. It was stressed again that he wouldn't be allowed home until satisfactory feeding had been established and until he had reached a viable weight. I then went to the sister of the premature unit to collect sterile bottles for my expressed milk.

Before leaving the hospital we decided we wanted to visit Will. The two of us stood forlornly over his cot looking at this tiny creature and both of us were in tears. Ed could not even bear to pick Will up. It was not that he rejected him, I knew that. I knew he was just feeling overwhelmed with pity for the tiny child whose life was to be so blighted. I gave Will a cuddle and cried.

We then left the hospital. I was in my slippers, nightdress and my mother's coat. Fortunately we got a taxi almost immediately and were soon home. My parents were wonderful in providing everything for us. They bought me some cigars – the brand I smoked. They made us tea, gave us whisky and generally looked after us. At our request they then left us, understanding that we wanted to be alone together.

It was an overwhelming future we felt we faced. At that point we were thinking in terms of the "rest of our lives". Another mother of a mongol child whom we met some months later confirmed, "Yes, one thinks big in those first few weeks". We thought big in those first few hours.

Both of us questioned "why has it happened to me?" Very fleetingly I thought why had he been born at all and that it would have been better if he hadn't. But by then I had so strongly related to Will, I loved him already too much for me to seriously wish him not born. At no point did either Ed or I think of rejecting Will. It just did not enter our heads or our hearts. We did not know then that parents could and did sometimes reject their child. We did not know that some parents leave their handicapped babies in hospital and leave other people to arrange care. We knew nothing about children who were not normal; nor did we know anything about their parents.

Besides "thinking big" in those first few hours, I also went through time and time again the events of the afternoon. That same mother who had told us about her reaction to the fact that her child was a mongol also remarked on how vividly, even thirteen years later, she remembered how she was told. Later, meeting other parents and reading the little literature there is on such matters, I found that the vivid memory is common. What is different is how people were told, when and what they were told and by whom. How parents find out that their child is handicapped is undoubtedly crucial to their acceptance or otherwise of the fact their child is handicapped.

At least parents of mongol children should not nowadays be kept waiting long for a diagnosis. Right from the outset we both felt sympathy for parents who had had to go through the long painful process of slowly realising that something was not quite right with their child. Mongolism can be diagnosed quite quickly and definitively. The presence of an extra chromosome in each cell, the cause of mongolism, can be confirmed by doing a chromosome analysis of the baby's cells.

Observable physical features and behaviour may be quite distinctive and lead a paediatrician to make a fairly confident diagnosis without checking it with a chromosome analysis. I am sure though that most would wish to confirm the diagnosis before committing themselves. On the other hand, the physical characteristics may not be very marked. Will's weren't very evident; even the sister of the premature unit said later she had not suspected it, although she had handled several mongol babies.

Looking back on how we were told, the main thing I resented was being told on my own. It was quite evident, or should have been, to those concerned at the hospital that although Ed and I were not married we were closely involved both with each other and with Will. Ed had been present at the birth, he had visited Will daily. I don't know whether the consultant even thought about it. My feeling is that either they just didn't consider us together or if they did they had decided that to pre-arrange a meeting to talk to both of us would have been to cause us fears based on wrong speculations. The other possibility was that the consultant, having just received the result of the test, wanted to tell me immediately and directly.

The latter he certainly did. I was told straight out that Will was a mongol, that mongolism was a condition for which there was no known cure, and that no known cure was even envisaged. I appreciated the directness. There is obviously no "nice" way to tell a mother of a new born baby that her baby is handicapped. Another thing I was later to appreciate was that the consultant did not tell me, as so many other parents of mongol children were told (and a few still are), that they should not expect their child ever to do anything. He left Will's potentialities quite open, basically by evading the issue. Another issue, which was not raised, was whether we would look after Will or put him into care. It was not a question for us since it simply did not enter our heads. However for some parents the question is put to them immediately with the warning that whichever decision they make they will have to live with for the rest of their lives. An impossible decision for a mother just after giving birth.

Whilst Will's potentialities were evaded, we were warned at the outset that mongolism was often accompanied by certain other congenital defects of heart and bowel, and that they also suffered from one or two other physical weaknesses. At the time we paid little attention to that information, feeling that we had quite enough to take in already. The consultant did keep saying to Ed and to me, when we were on our own or together, "Are there any more questions you want to ask, please don't hesitate to ask about anything?" Whilst it made us feel we could ask questions, since we didn't know anything about mongolism, we didn't know what questions to ask.

Our experience, of little information being initially proferred, seems common. It would appear that consultants tell parents so little for a variety of reasons. Firstly, the medical profession assume that a little knowledge to a lay person is a dangerous thing and therefore it is better to tell nothing at all, and failing that tell only the bare essentials. Secondly, I got the feeling that they didn't think we could "take" any more information. Finally, although paediatricians may be well versed in the physical problems associated with mongolism they are concerned only with the child's physical well-being and not with the potential of the child's whole being. The child's body is thus conveniently divorced, for medical purposes, from its human social context. My comments are generalisations about the medical profession drawn from my experience. There are many who obviously do not fit into this standard attitude. But since the medical profession at the consultant level is predominantly white and male, are drawn from the middle class, and have all been schooled and practice in the same medical system, it is not surprising that one can make generalisations. We did meet one or two who overtly or just through natural instinct challenged that system. They were to be a great source of strength and support to us.

4. LIMBO LAND

For the first few days after we had been told about Will we were much as we had been that first evening – dazed and shocked. Ed stayed off work and apart from visiting Will in hospital we did little. We had a shopping expedition and I bought a very expensive knitted skirt and jacket. Ed read voraciously, mainly detective novels, but I found I could not concentrate on anything. I watched television, at least stared at the television set but took in little of what I saw. Often I would realise that I had been staring for some time and could not even tell what programme I was watching.

Not surprisingly certain sights and sounds triggered off our fears for our child and our future. I remember one morning finding Ed in tears. At the bottom of our garden on the other side of a high wall is the playground of a primary school. At 10.45 a.m. each weekday morning during term time there is a sudden burst of sound, children screaming, shouting and generally letting off steam, normal children, playing normally at a normal school. The thought that our child might never do those things was very hurtful. Equally hard was seeing children, normal children and babies, and having to realise that one would never walk down the street with Will in quite the same way.

Of course in those early days we remained incredibly ignorant about mongolism. The hospital had told us very little, we had asked for little further information and no-one so far had been forthcoming with any. From the outset we wanted our friends and relatives to know that Will was a mongol. My parents told our relatives and one or two of our friends, and we asked that the word be passed round. I feared the telephone calls of people phoning up to congratulate me on having a baby and then having to say "but he's a mongol". In fact that happened only once with a close friend, although of course we had to tell many people about him at different stages. One of the first people we talked to was my brother-in-law, who is a doctor. He provided a good balance between sympathy and information. Following that first tentative step out into the world as parents of a handicapped child, we then slowly made contact with our other friends.

The most frequent thing said and written to us in those early days was, "they're usually very loving and affectionate children". It was said by people meaning well, but I reacted quite violently against what I regarded as a sop which I felt was being offered to me as a substitute for a normal child. Like so many other attitudes it was one which I was to reappraise fundamentally later. Most people did not know how to respond to us. They did not know what to say, but usually once we began to talk they would follow our lead. However, some people deliberately avoided the whole subject as if we hadn't had a baby, yet we knew they knew. It was both hurtful to us and hard since it was the subject uppermost in our minds and we both found relief in talking about it.

Ed spent the whole of that week at home and we barely parted from each other's company. We developed a sensitivity to each other's moods. One would sense when the other was needing reassurance or just a hug and usefully one was normally feeling strong when the other was weak. I was certainly the more weepy. I was still weak and fairly tired from giving birth. My recovery had not been helped by the emotional strain.

Each day we visited the hospital twice. The first visit or two we found painful but soon we found that when we were actually with Will we were more concerned about trying to encourage him to suck, or in learning how to bath him or in just watching him, than in the fact that he was abnormal. It also soon became obvious that it would be quite a long haul before Will could come home. A few weeks at least, we reckoned, although the doctors would never commit themselves. They would just say "Don't worry, we'll let you know when he's ready". Given the length of time Will would probably have to stay in we decided it was best if Ed returned to work and then took some more time off when Will came out of hospital, so that Will could start life at home with both of us. So after a week together, Ed returned to work. His first morning back was difficult. He was asked by more than one person "What are you going to do with him?" The first time he did not initially understand the question. It then dawned on him that what was implied was whether we were intending to keep Will or not. It was the first time the question was put directly to either of us and since the question had not entered either of our heads it was not surprising that Ed did not understand it. It was also extremely hurtful to be asked, as the parent of a new born baby, whether you intend to keep him. No-one directly asked me the question but that in itself is a sad reflection on the way that society assumes that fathers of new born babies are less concerned and have less love for their child than the mother.

With Ed back at work I was left in a strange limbo land. My baby was in hospital. I was at home. Somehow I managed to fill the days. I went shopping and bought all the baby things I had not got round to buying before his birth. I scoured the shops for the smallest sized baby clothes I could find. My mother bought some size "o" baby vests which looked as though they were meant for dolls, but even those were too big for him. Besides pottering round on domestic jobs and seeing friends most of my time was taken up with visiting the hospital and with starting the difficult task of trying to find out as much about mongolism as I could.

I visited the hospital twice daily and continued trying to feed Will. The longer the struggle went on the harder it became, not helped by the fact that my milk was slowly drying up. The endless expressing of my milk was becoming an ordeal. I had none of the pleasure of breast-feeding, only the continual tedious milking of myself. It was not surprising it virtually dried up. One day I took a bottle into the hospital with a tiny amount of milk in the bottom. I handed it to a nurse and she abruptly said "Is that all?" It was a crushing blow. To that point the only thing I could do for Will was to give him my milk. I could not directly feed him, most of his care was done by the nurses and the giving of milk was for me a tangible bond. My only contribution. That nurse nearly broke it. After another futile attempt to feed Will I drove home feeling terribly depressed. I sat half way up the stairs and cried. I felt a total failure. I'd failed to produce a normal child; "almost anyone can produce a normal child," I thought, "but I can't and I can't even feed him."

Fortunately, when I next saw the registrar he was very reassuring. Although I did not quite believe him he told me that as long as my milk kept being produced, even in the tiniest quantities, when the demand was there, that is when Will began to suck, the supply would increase to meet the demand. I kept going, helped too by the nurses, who were mostly gentle and sympathetic. One or two were particularly helpful and I knew that they were offering me special support.

It was partially my fierce determination not to be defeated and partially the support in the unit and of Ed that I persisted. The desire to feed him became much more than my original romantic idea of motherhood. It was to do with being determined that my child, who had started with so little, was going to have everything I could give him.

During those three weeks that I was at home without Will, trying to find out about mongolism proved as hard as trying to breast feed him. In our search we had little assistance from any professional person. I had a visit at home from my health visitor, who was kindly and sympathetic but openly admitted that she knew virtually nothing about mongolism. She did leave me two short pamphlets to read. They were so bad that we would have done better not to read them. Their main message was one of doom and gloom. They offered no practical advice about anything we could do but just warned us of all the things our child would not do. They warned that our child would not crawl until two, walk until four, or talk until seven – that is if he achieved any speech at all. There were lists of probable physical problems we might face, like colds, bad circulation, skin problems, obesity, congenital defects as well as mental retardation. A few comments as to how "loving and affectionate" mongol children are were added to compensate for the bad news.

Apart from that one visit from the health visitor no-one else in that first period, no social worker, doctor, nurse or organisation approached us to give us any more information about mongolism or even put us in touch with anyone who might help. The one exception was that the health visitor told me that the National Society for Mentally Handicapped Children ran a counselling service for parents of handicapped children. I made an appointment to see a counsellor and both of us went. It was a bizarre session. We had a lengthy argument with the counsellor about the importance or otherwise of literacy which stemmed from a comment I made that I found it hard to accept the prospect that my child would be illiterate. It was helpful being just able to talk to a sympathetic listener about our fears and our reactions but we were looking for concrete help and advice, not just sympathy. We left feeling that we hadn't really moved forward in understanding the problems we and our child would face.

A few days later I returned to the National Society for Mentally Handicapped Children and scoured their bookshop for any relevant literature. I found a little, but once again nothing that was of any concrete help. The social, medical, and physical information given in those short pamphlets was unsatisfactory. The medical information was so simplified that it mystified as much as it clarified. Very little was said about social problems and even less about where or to whom you could go. Advice as to what you could do was non-existent. Sometimes reading things would upset me. Something suddenly would bring home to me my child's handicap and I would burst into tears. Living in limbo with Will in hospital and me at home left me a lot of time to think and to try to come to terms with my child's handicap.

While I feel critical of the hospital for the little information they gave us I realise, in retrospect, that their attitude was positive. They did stress treating Will as a normal child. Throughout his stay in hospital they maintained their initial position of not stating what his potential might be and in stating so little they left a lot open. Their attitude became quite clear when I talked to the registrar about the kind of problems I might face when I took Will home. I also asked him whether there was anything special I should do because of his mongolism. "No, nothing special", was the reply. "Just treat him as normal". He told me "He'll need feeding and loving and playing with just like a normal child". That attitude had been obviously integral to the whole way they had encouraged me to treat Will from the outset. I appreciated the fact that they stressed that my child should be treated as a normal child and yet by doing that they were ignoring the special treatment that later I found out a mongol child needs. A mongol child is not normal, it needs special treatment and with special treatment it will be more normal. But that was to come later.

Fortunately, despite the lack of information, I just instinctively felt that Will should be encouraged to do anything a normal child should do. Partly this was tied up with my initial reaction to the fact that my child was handicapped. Needless to say my "reaction" was really a complex, and in some ways contradictory, set of reactions. My hospital records, read illicitly, state something to the effect "Was very upset but took it very sensibly". In one sense, I suppose, the report was relatively true. I was visibly very upset but also in their terms "sensible". I did not have hysterics or want to kill myself or my baby. I did not reject Will or refuse to accept the situation.

But the hospital report tells only a tiny part of the story. To have to come to terms with the fact that one's own flesh and blood, grown in one's own womb, is not normal is to have to come to terms with many things within oneself. It is an enormously humbling experience. In one stroke all those conscious and subconscious fantasies parents have for their children were knocked to the ground. Whilst Will was still in the incubator, before we knew of his mongolism, I remember Ed looking at one of his tiny feet and joking about how that foot might be the foot which scored the winning goal for Arsenal in a cup final twenty odd years hence. It was the kind of comment half joking, half fanciful, part wishing, that parents make, particularly of tiny babies. In the first few weeks after we knew about Will's handicap it was the kind of comment we did not make. We were painfully aware of all the things he definitely would not do. It left little room for us to fantasise about greatness and glory.

Even more basically we had to realise that not only

would Will not score the winning goal in a cup final, but that he might not be able to do the most basic things parents assume their children will be able to do. A friend commented one evening on how he had hoped that by encouraging his kid to write on the walls of his own room he could discourage him from writing on other walls. He was explaining how it didn't work and of how the kid kept writing on all the walls. He then finished the description by saying "Just you wait". Ed commented "It'd be great if Will did write on the walls". There was an uncomfortable silence. We were having to assimilate the possible limitations of our child.

Although humbled, my pride played a part in my many-sided reaction to Will's mongolism. He was my child. I loved him, I was proud of him and society was going to have to accept him. This was not a reaction I was very aware of at first, but in embryo it was certainly there. It was to manifest itself much more strongly later. However proud and humbled we were one reaction Ed and I did not have was to feel ashamed or guilty. We never thought to try to conceal his mongolism. This was made easier for us as neither of us had any religious or other form of belief in the "sins of the fathers", "reincarnation", the "will of God" or the will of any other supernatural power. We both knew that it was simply a genetic accident, the result of Will having an extra chromosome.

But whilst I accepted it and did not feel guilty, I did feel a failure. These two reactions may well seem contradictory and in many respects they are. If I had followed my logical response to the scientific reason for mongolism it should have led me to realise that neither Ed nor I had any control over the presence or otherwise of an extra chromosome and therefore I should not have felt either success or failure about it.

My initial reactions were obviously conditioned partly

by my ignorance, partly by my own nature but largely by the dominant attitude of society towards handicapped people. Later, as I found out more, I changed many of my attitudes. My feelings towards Will never changed, but I did lose my sense of failure. The more I learnt about and experienced the attitude of society towards handicapped children, and, even worse, handicapped adults, the more I realised that the failure was the society that we live in and not me. My feeling turned into one of anger. But the change took time and in those early weeks I was still just trying to come to terms with the new world we found ourselves confronting, a world of normality and abnormality.

Right from the first conversations we had with people we felt that a lid was being lifted off a whole area of society of which we had been barely aware. Neither of us had really had any contact with handicapped children or adults. I dimly remembered a boy who lived down the road from us when I was a child who was "not quite normal", and went to a special school. When the boy grew up his parents moved to a farm on the edge of the moors so that their son could have meaningful work. I remember my parents saying how much they admired his parents. Yet suddenly, in talking with people, we found that almost everyone had had experience of handicapped relatives or friends. People had aunts, cousins, sisters or brothers who were handicapped. They too remembered the child down the road or the old man in the village who was not quite normal. We became aware that we were not the only people in the world who had a handicapped child.

My three weeks of living in limbo came to an end when I decided to move back into the hospital to make a final effort to try and establish the feeding of Will. The first three days were a disaster. The registrar managed to get me a single room in which I could stay, on the main maternity floor, a whole floor away from the safe and sympathetic confines of the premature unit. I was put there with Will and, largely, left alone to try to feed my child. It was a nightmare. What he didn't take from the breast, virtually his whole meal, I then had to spoon feed to him. Meals took well over an hour. I got tired, distraught, and what I had been looking forward to, actually being with my baby for the first time, turned into horror. It was compounded by the day sister apparently trying to sabotage the whole experiment. She obviously resented this interruption to the normal running of her wards. Fortunately the registrar was determined the experiment would work. He managed to move me to a single room almost opposite the special unit so that I could have Will in my room or feed him in the unit, where I had sympathetic care and help. I could also leave Will in the unit when I wanted a babysitter so I had the chance of a break or two from the hospital. It meant Ed and I could go out for a meal together in the evenings. I also went to the dentist, where I burst into tears telling him about Will, and I made my first "public" appearance: I went to a press conference for the launching of a report on Discrimination against Women in the Film and Television Industry, which had been drawn up by my union. It was an uncomfortable experience making my first steps out into the world as a very self-conscious parent of a handicapped child.

From the moment I moved down to the room opposite the unit things improved daily. Slowly Will began to learn to suck. He was test weighed at each feed and slowly his daily intake from me went up. I felt ten feet tall, helped to grow in stature by all the nurses who would congratulate me every time we broke a former "quantity" record. The day Will actually sucked from me the equivalent of his full amount for a feed everyone seemed genuinely thrilled. That was the moment when the registrar told me Will could go home.

At that time no-one told me that mongol children have particular difficulty in sucking, that they even find sucking a bottle hard, so the combination of a mongol premature baby provided pretty formidable problems to overcome in establishing breast feeding. But from the outset I was determined that Will would do what other children did. If other premature babies could learn to breast feed, Will could. In the process of learning to suck he also had to learn to cry for food. He would have died from starvation in those first few weeks if anyone had waited for him to cry with hunger before feeding him. By the time I took him home from hospital he had both learnt to cry for food and to suck from the breast. The latter achievement showed he could already do something "the books" said he could not do.

I was absolutely thrilled to take Will home. I felt like any proud mum. After six weeks he was put in clothes for the first time and, escorted by a nurse, Ed and I carried Will out of the hospital. We drove home excited, nervous, and thrilled to be taking our baby home at last.

5. AT HOME

Once at home, Will, Ed and I could try to work out our lives together in the same way that any other parents have to do. Initially we followed our instincts and the advice from the registrar at the hospital to treat Will normally, but since he was our first child it was a little difficult for us to know what that meant. At one level he did need treating like other babies: feeding, changing, washing and cuddling. At another level he was not quite normal. For a start he was so tiny; even first size clothes were large on him, and because he was so tiny one felt he was very delicate. More worrying was that whilst he fed normally, and during that first week at home he registered a massive weight gain, it was evident he was a very undemanding child. Although he had learnt to cry when he was hungry he often did not demand a meal and there were occasions when he still fell asleep on the job. The work of sucking was still enormously tiring for him. However, at that early stage we just felt triumphant that he had learnt to suck and that he had begun to grow and become stronger.

Slowly also I began to relax, my confidence growing as he grew. I relaxed further as he showed no signs of repeating a "blue" attack which he had had in hospital. It had happened a few days before we brought him home and had given me a bad fright. I was feeding him one day and looked down to find that he had turned a deep blue from head to foot. Quickly I stood up and looked round the unit in panic for someone to help me. There was a nurse in there but she was tube feeding another baby and could not put it down. Fortunately in the other section of the unit, separated by a glass panel, the sister was free and happened to look through at that moment. She moved fast. It was very impressive to see the confident, assertive but speedy way in which she took over the situation. Immediately she reached for the oxygen mask which was above his cot and for a tube to suck out his throat in case he was choking. Quite quickly he returned to a "normal" colour. The doctor, of course, was immediately called and Will was given an ECG. To our relief they could find no evidence of anything serious that could have caused the attack. But in fact that episode was the writing on the wall. None of us realised it at the time and, whilst I was frightened of such an attack happening again, I did not think it was a symptom of anything more important. Such blueness did not return again for some months, and when it did we were at least partially informed of its cause.

Because of Will's essentially undemanding nature he was a very easy baby. As soon as the doctor thought he was large enough to go through the night without a feed it was dropped and he did not complain. In fact he rarely complained. He cried only when there was some obvious discomfort. Because he was so undemanding one had to feel his needs. Much to our relief, it was evident that nothing was wrong with his senses. Quite quickly it became clear that he could see and focus on things. He responded to sounds quite positively, loving music, being frightened of loud sharp sounds and responding to the human voice, particularly mine and Ed's. Although he did not show signs of being precocious in early movement, such as holding his head up unsupported, he was not a particularly "floppy" baby. We had been led to expect that he would be from "the literature" we had read about mongol babies.

Those first few weeks at home were very much like the first few weeks of any parents with their first baby. We had to adjust our routine, become used to leaving our bedroom door open at night, and tune our ears into listening for baby sounds. I had to face being house-bound and baby-bound, my mobility being very restricted both by having a baby and by the fact that we felt, after six weeks in the special care unit, he needed a few weeks at home before we started taking him out and about. Even more we had to confront having a third party entering into what had been an exclusive twosome. It was a difficult adjustment but one made easier by the fact that Will was so unintrusive.

Most of our friends and relatives appeared to accept Will unhesitatingly. Many were keen too to show their support of us. However, we did get some surprises. People did not necessarily react as I might have predicted they would. Some people emerged as particularly open to him and to us about it all and some recoiled from it and almost pretended nothing had happened or that Will was normal. By and large Will was utterly spoilt and since he was unaware of it, it was, in a sense, we parents who were being spoilt. Many presents were sent or given to him, many from people whom we knew were making a gesture of solidarity. There were others who had obviously chosen a present much more carefully than they might have done and that again we read as a gesture of support and welcomed it. I can still remember almost every present that was given to Will, who gave it, and the "strengthening" effect it had on us. Will also benefited. He had lovely mobiles to watch, toys to play with, clothes to wear, shawls to keep him warm, and a beautiful red wool carpet for his room which my mother gave him, anticipating the day when he could play on it.

It helped us that people accepted Will. It was a good

start but I feared that it would not always be the case and that it would be something that I would have to fight for. My reaction was a reflection of my fierce love and pride. I always took the trouble to see that he was "well dressed", that he had nice clothes and was always clean in every way. It was my way of saying to the world "here is *my* child, I am proud of him". I also recognised that if I wanted him to be accepted I would have to do my part in encouraging his development as much as possible, but that society would have to do its part in recognising and accepting his limitations.

In those first few weeks at home I established a relationship with one doctor which was to be of crucial importance to me for the rest of Will's life. Before I brought Will home from the hospital the registrar at St A's explained that St A's had a "Home Care Unit" which was staffed by a doctor, a sister and a secretary. He never really described the function of the unit but said that since I lived in the St A's area, he would, if I wished, ask if Will could be put on the list of the unit so that during the weeks immediately after Will had been released from hospital he would be visited at home to check that everything was going smoothly. Being nervous of taking Will home I quickly said that I would welcome such visits.

The day before I took Will home there was a knock on my hospital room door and a small woman, apparently Indian (I later found out she was from Sri Lanka) came in and introduced herself as Dr Z from the Home Care Unit. She asked if I minded her asking a few questions about Will. She questioned me about his birth, feeding and other problems. She then asked me what my plans were for when I took him home. I explained that for the first week Ed would be at home too, so that I should be able to cope with practical problems. I also explained that I was very nervous. After six weeks of always having professionals on hand for help and advice the prospect of being on my own frightened me. Dr Z then asked when I would like visiting at home. The question rather surprised me. Most doctors tell you when and whether they will visit you. She then rather tentatively said "I don't want to intrude on you and your husband during your first week at home with William". Quickly I said "Oh, you wouldn't be intruding, I'd be very relieved if you would come at the end of the week just to check up on everything". We agreed she should call on the Friday and she left.

For the first time in my experience a doctor had actually shown real sensitivity about a human, family situation. It impressed me deeply. Later many more things about Dr Z were to impress me. On that Friday she visited me, weighed Will, questioned me about his behaviour, listened to his heart and breathing and declared him "doing very well". We didn't talk much but she handled Will gently and with obvious care. She made a few very supportive remarks about how good she thought it was for Will that he was being breast fed. We didn't at that first visit discuss his mongolism but rather gently felt out the situation. During those first few weeks at home she visited him once a week on average to give him a routine check up. I was given the number of the Home Care Unit and told I could phone any week day if I was worried. Only twice in the first few weeks did I have need to. The first time he had slight bleeding from the bowel which panicked me but on investigation didn't prove to be anything serious. The second time I called because Will had been crying without obvious cause all the previous evening. Dr Z came, examined him and could find absolutely nothing wrong. I felt guilty that I had called her out for nothing. She was so reassuring, so understanding, explaining that she too was a mother of a small child and had also experienced the worries of a baby crying for no particular reason that I ceased to feel guilty or silly. She also stressed that if I was worried I should *never* feel inhibited about calling the Unit.

My breakthrough in getting information about mongolism came about quite accidentally. Someone I knew at the BBC phoned me for some information. I gave it to her and she then asked if I had had my baby. It was one of those occasions when I had then to decide whether I would tell her that he was a mongol. She was not someone I knew well, but someone I bumped into from time to time. I decided to explain that he was a mongol. She immediately replied "How extraordinary". I was a little taken aback by her remark. I had had a variety of replies or embarrassed silences or evasions, but never such an immediate registration of something rather out of the ordinary. She then went on to explain that she had recently been working for a programme about handicapped children, had visited various schools and organisations involved with them, and perhaps I would like her to send me any information she had about mongolism and organisations concerned with mentally handicapped children. She sent me a pile of material, in which was included the address of an organisation called the Down's Babies Association. Down's Syndrome is the proper medical term for mongolism, and is derived from Dr Landon Down, who first described the syndrome about a hundred years ago. It was only comparatively recently, however, some twenty years ago, that the cause – an extra chromosome – was discovered.

My friend also told me that someone else, someone whom in fact I knew quite well, had recently been working on a programme for the handicapped on ITV. She suggested I contact him as he would probably know even more about the subject. I immediately phoned him and he recommended that I should get in touch right away with the Down's Babies Association, saying that he thought they would be of great help to us. He gave me their address and also the phone number of the man who founded and was the leading force behind the association, Rex Brinkworth.

A little tentatively I phoned Rex Brinkworth but no sooner had he answered and I had explained who I was and why I was phoning than I realised I had no need to be tentative. His response was like a wind of hope and support blowing down the phone. Firstly he asked me at great length and with obvious great interest all about Will's life to date, his prematurity, his feeding, his development and about his general health. He also asked me how we had been told, how the doctors had treated us and if we had had any other help. For the first time I felt I was talking to someone who really knew about Down's Syndrome. At last I was getting more than just sympathy and support. I was getting information from someone who knew both most of what there was to know about Down's Syndrome and also what was not known. It was also obvious that he was not concerned with the child just as a "medical", "sociological", "educational", or "statistical" phenomenon, but with the whole child and its immediate environment.

During our phone conversation Rex Brinkworth told me that the association gave parents "training schedules", which covered almost every aspect of early training, stimulation and diet of Down's Syndrome babies. He stressed that we could not start too young stimulating Will and urged me to join the association. With no hesitation I agreed to send the modest subscription. But a doctor's letter, he explained, was necessary before the association would send me a copy of their training schedules, since some of their advice, such as that on diet, would be better followed in conjunction with one's own doctor's knowledge and acceptance. I knew there would be no trouble in asking Dr Z for a letter but I decided to use the request for a letter as a reason for going to my own GP to register Will and to make contact with him about my child. Whilst I hoped that the

Home Care Unit would continue to care for him I did not know how long we would be able to benefit from that arrangement; also they did not operate at nights or during weekends.

My mother baby-sat for me whilst I went to see my GP. When I arrived I found that the surgery already had voluminous information/records on Will, which had been sent to them from the hospital. I explained that I wished to register my baby, but my doctor showed absolutely no interest in Will's particular handicap, his prematurity or his development. I then said that I had heard of an association for parents of Down's Syndrome babies. I told him that they sent parents training schedules and briefly explained both these and the letter of consent requested from one's GP. He had not heard of the association, did not enquire further about it but scribbled a note to them in accordance with my request. I thanked him and then began to mutter something about possible other physical/medical problems which Down's Syndrome children frequently had. He quickly shut me up by standing up as if to denote the "audience" was over and just said "Oh well, there are some very good hospitals in London". I left his surgery in tears of frustration and outrage.

It still seems to me absolutely monstrous that a doctor can devote less than ten minutes of his time and considerably less than ten minutes of his concern to one of his patients who is registering her two month old mentally handicapped child who had been born prematurely and who would almost certainly present quite serious medical, physical and emotional problems. My response was to change doctors instantly, but I never wrote to the one I left explaining why I left. At the time, feeling as I did and still do when I recall it, an uncontrollable anger towards him, there was no way that I could write a coherent letter. My new GP was quite different. As things worked out he saw little of

Will, but from the outset he was interested in him – for instance, when I registered him he insisted that I should bring Will so that he could examine him and meet him. Thinking about my experience with the first GP, what made me even more angry was the thought of what other parents do, faced with an equally unresponsive, unsympathetic GP. I had had Dr Z from the Home Care Unit; I know how one changes one's GP; I live in an area of London where there is considerable choice of GP; I have a brother and a brother-in-law in the medical profession available to give me advice. In short I faced my particular problem from a very privileged position. I often thought, and still do, of people, possibly single-parent families, facing the emotional, social and physical problems a handicapped child presents, without sympathetic support from their doctor.

When Will was two months old I took him to the hospital for his first "check up" by the consultant. At that visit everything appeared to be well. Looking back on it there was in fact a signal of what was to come, but no-one at the time took any notice of it. The consultant gave Will a once-over examination and asked us questions about his development. There were two students with him and both were asked to examine him and listen to his heart. The consultant asked them what they heard. The male student said he could hear nothing abnormal; the female student said she thought she could hear a murmur. The consultant said he had heard nothing abnormal but listened again, his second listening confirming his initial one. Whilst at the hospital Will had a chest X-ray, something he always hated, and he screamed all the time he was strapped to that cold machinery with his arms held up above his head. We returned home feeling reassured, the chest X-ray having been the only traumatic part of the visit, but also none the wiser about Down's Syndrome, the hospital having given us no more advice or information.

Fortunately we were not to be left in our comparative ignorance for long. The material from the Down's Babies Association arrived virtually by return of post. I read it all instantly and avidly, later going through it more slowly. There was a booklet called "Improving Babies with Down's Syndrome", written by Rex Brinkworth and Dr Joseph Collins. In it they both gave their overall aims, that of improving the potential of Down's Syndrome children, and also gave fairly detailed advice and information as to how that could be achieved. That advice was supplemented by the more specific training schedules.

The training schedules were broken down into three stages from birth to five years. It was stressed that you cannot start too young in beginning the special care and stimulation that a Down's Syndrome baby needs. Each aspect of the child's physical and mental needs and development were covered and advice given as to what could be done to help. For the baby from birth to six months old, advice was given on feeding, the need for warmth and improving the baby's circulation and skin. It was not only reassuring finally to understand why I had had such great problems teaching Will to suck, but also to understand what the problems might be and how we might overcome them when he started on solid foods. The advice on skin care I also immediately followed, hoping that by starting on the right path we might later avoid problems.

As important, was the advice they gave for early sensory training. The schedule explained: "The young mongol baby is generally ill-developed, especially in its nervous system and circulation. It is usually limp and unresponsive; its muscles appear completely soft and powerless and it rarely cries or demands anything."

Unlike the other literature we had read, this state of affairs was not regarded as something which had to be lived with but as a problem to be worked on. To help the muscles they gave advice and described exercises which should be given daily, even to a tiny baby. The exercises were designed both to stimulate and improve mobility. The same theory was applied to the development of the baby's other senses and again they gave advice as to how that could be done. Behind all the advice was the theory that since everything about a Down's Syndrome baby is ill-developed, slow and sluggish, you need to give it extra stimulation in every way.

It was on that theory that all the schedules were based. The training and treatment of a five year old was not radically different from that for a small baby, though obviously the exercises, diet, sensory stimulation and so on were gradually developed to meet the needs of the growing child.

It was a great release to me to read the booklet and the training schedules. At last I had something which didn't approach the fact of having a mentally handicapped child as a tragedy but as a reality of life, a problem, but one which could be better faced with the support of others. It was also seen as a problem which could be, at least, partially solved. Suddenly here was someone telling me of all the things I could do *for* my child and explaining *why* they needed doing and what the effect would be. Instead of reading lists of all the things which we should expect our child not to do and of all the physical and mental problems we could expect, here was someone saying "we do not know what your child's potential is but it is almost certainly much greater than those about you have probably led you to expect". The message was a very long way from the old attitude handed out by lay people and professionals alike: "your child won't do anything" – an attitude which tended to become a self-fulfilling prophecy.

At last I could do something positive to help modify my child's handicap. Will was given a ten minute work out of exercises every day. After every bath, his skin was rubbed with a rough towel and then with lanolin cream to help his circulation and keep his skin soft. From that point on Will was *never* allowed to lie in his cot staring awake at a blank ceiling. If he didn't have company to play with him, talk to him or sing to him, he was surrounded by sensory stimulation – music, mobiles, and simple toys that made noises. Everything needed to be a lot larger than life, or very simple so that he could respond with the minimum requirement of strength and skill. In fact one of the things he found endlessly fascinating was a "mobile" which I hung up in the kitchen. It was one of those Christmas decorations – a twirly tinsel affair that was bright red and blue on one side and silver on the other. It twirled with the slightest current of air, sparkled with even a tiny amount of light and so was endlessly colourful, bright and in motion. The perfect mobile and cheap. Another of his first toys which gave him endless delight was a sheet of greaseproof paper. Very quickly he found he could grasp it, wave it about and make a nice crackly noise.

The other message explicit and implicit in all the material from the Down's Babies Association was that Down's Syndrome babies and children should be accepted and recognised as part of the community, the onus initially being on the parents to accept their child as part of the family but also on the community to accept the child as part of it. The association said parents "must take their babies out into the world. Mongol children should see people and be seen by people. In this way mothers can teach others that a handicapped child can lead a meaningful life". It was reinforcing for me to see other people saying what I thought and believed. The association also sent round a regular newsletter which, besides giving handy hints and information about the organisation, also made one aware that there were many other parents who were fighting for the rights of their child to be part of society. Later I found out that the association also operated as a pressure group able to formulate informed demands on behalf of the educational, social and medical needs of Down's Syndrome children.

6. SETTLING DOWN

What with one thing and another it was some time before I settled down to really work out my life with Will at home. Not only had I to adjust to having a baby at home, I also had to work out just what particular care and attention Will needed. Slowly I did become more confident and stopped popping in to look at him all the time whilst he was asleep just to make sure he was all right. As Will put on weight we also felt less need to cosset him so much. I began taking him out and about and we both took him with us when we went out in the evenings to see friends. We even managed to get out on our own once or twice. Usually my mother baby-sat as we did not feel we could leave him with someone who was not experienced with babies or whom we did not have confidence in. The first film we went to see was sadly memorable, not because it was a great film but because of one line in it together with the audience's reaction. The film was *Shampoo* and at one point in it the character played by Goldie Hawn was trying to persuade her boyfriend to marry her. She argued that she wanted to have children, was getting older, turned thirty and that if she didn't have a baby quickly she might have a "mongoloid idiot". The audience laughed.

Ed had to make only minor adjustments to his routine. He had turned down a series of evening lectures but otherwise his work pattern followed the normal working week. Five days a week he left the house just after nine in the morning and returned at about seven in the evening. It left him little time for contact with Will during the week. However, at the weekend he would spend much time playing, cuddling, handling and changing his nappies and once Will started on solids he would often feed him. It was clear that during periods when Ed was in close contact with Will he was much more interested and excited by him than during those times when he was to see little of him apart from a good-night cuddle.

In contrast (to Ed) my life had changed radically. I was at home most of the time with the primary child care resting in my hands. I was very tied, partly from my own commitment and partly because Will did need more care than a normal baby. The struggle to breast feed him had been so great that I couldn't risk his having "the odd bottle" which would have given me a break but might have undermined the well-established breast feeding routine.

Curiously, for the most part I did not resent my tied situation and also contrary to my expectations I did not find that by having a baby my life had come to an end. I found, as in so many other situations, that it was a case of trying to minimise the time spent on things I didn't enjoy.

The aspect of being at home all the time that I didn't enjoy and from time to time resented was the fact that the main burden of domestic labour fell on me. We tried to work out a division of labour but my presence at home inevitably meant that I did most of the shopping, cooking and cleaning. Every now and again I would complain and demand that Ed should do an increased share. He would then have a burst of energy and do a certain amount but things would slowly slip as he got caught up in his work commitments. However, the child care aspect of being at home I never resented. Much to my surprise I found that I thoroughly enjoyed looking after Will, feeding him, changing him, playing with him and just endlessly watching him. It did sadden me that Ed saw so relatively little of Will but there seemed no way out of the problem. One of us had to work full time to earn the primary family wage and our respective jobs were not compatible with an arrangement by which we could both work part time and share the child care part time. At that stage I did not want to go out to work and leave Will, nor did I feel that I could.

I had anticipated the problem before Will's birth. I had been in the middle of writing a history book and had completed most of the research before his birth so that I could write it up at home whilst my baby slept. This plan had been thrown by the fact that for some time my life was neither organised enough nor was my mind capable of concentration. But finally I did get things organised and wrote whilst he slept. I found having him very good discipline. He slept in the mornings and I knew that when I put him down at about ten I then had two to three hours to write. In the old days I would have made myself a cup of coffee, made a phone call or two, wandered round the garden and generally wasted time evading confronting the typewriter. With Will and his time limit I would sit down immediately he went to sleep and work.

I found it a great mental break to spend a part of each day thinking about something other than my own problems. It also made me feel less trapped, for although I remained physically home bound I no longer felt mentally confined. It was much harder trying to re-establish even a vestige of life outside the home than it was to re-establish my writing. All my commitments to other things outside were impossible to keep going except that I tried to keep up with some of my trade union activities. I was at the time a member of the executive of my union, representing freelance television members, and I did manage to get to quite a number of executive meetings. Ed encouraged me to continue going to the meetings and would make a special point of ensuring that he could look after Will. He thought it was important for me to maintain some contact with the world I had been involved in and with the world I hoped to actively re-join at some point. There were times when I felt that going out to a meeting was too much trouble and effort and I can well understand why women with babies retreat into their homes.

It is, and was, very hard for me to separate out my reactions to having a child from those which came from having a handicapped child. They were obviously not separate but equally they were not entirely the same. One mother wrote that parents, mothers in particular, tend to react to the news that their child is handicapped by either rejecting it or in finding their "mother love" is working overtime. Mine worked overtime and kept working overtime . . . It was equally hard for me to separate out the reactions of other people to me, to me as a mother, and to me as a mother of a handicapped child.

Having a child certainly re-defined me in people's eyes; having a handicapped child was an extension of that re-definition. I was very aware of a new attitude, not so much amongst close friends and relatives but more amongst people I knew less well and who knew me in a particular role. Mainly it emerged amongst people in my trade union where I was known as a woman who had fought for "women's rights". Whilst not a firebrand feminist, (I was always too shy to be such even if I had politically agreed with it) I was certainly identified, and didn't mind being so, as a "women's liberationist" and to many members of the union therefore suspect. But being pregnant had made me, in their eyes, more of a woman. There was an attitude that these "women's libbers" weren't really women at all and that the main way that they weren't really women was that they didn't have children. Actually being a mother and the mother of a handicapped child as well as continuing to fight for the equal rights of women caused people to re-evaluate their reaction to me. Undoubtedly I became regarded as a much more "serious" person now that I had become a "mother". Funnily enough it was a new role which I didn't immediately recognise. It was about four weeks after Will was born when I was living in hospital trying to feed him that the registrar said one day that I could come and go from the hospital as I pleased: "After all" he explained "you're not a patient, you're a mother". It was like being knocked on the head with an amazing bit of information about myself. "Christ, I'm a mother" I thought to myself, an entirely new role in life from any other I had had. At that moment I did not realise just how much that new role would affect how people would respond to me.

During the settling down period, which became a few months of relative calm and routine, we also had to come to terms with Will's handicap and what our possible future might be. We realised that however well he developed he would always be to some degree dependent on us. One of our immediate worries, a worry that is common to all parents of handicapped children whom they care for, was about how we could provide for Will in the event of our deaths. Ed made enquiries about his pension and arranged for it to go to Will if he were to die. We also wondered how else we could ensure that in the event of our deaths Will could be provided for so that at least he could be assured of a level of material care. The information from the Down's Babies Association had reinforced my belief that Will's potential was much greater than others had directly or indirectly implied. It made me believe that Will, with the right stimulation, help and extra help, could achieve a measure of independence, but I never believed he would be an entirely independent adult. Whilst it is very questionable what exactly an "independent adult" is, it is undoubtedly true that minimal literacy, numeracy, mechanical competence and coherent speech are basic requirements for an adult to "get about" in society.

Facing the prospect of Will's handicap and accepting it meant we could talk about it. Our openness was rewarded in the amount of feedback and information we received, the feedback coming both from the support and help of our friends and relatives and from professional organisations. Besides the advice and information we had received from the Down's Babies Association which I continued to act on daily we were also contacted through the National Society for Mentally Handicapped Children, to ask us if we would like to take part in a project at the Institute of Psychiatry. This was a series of one evening a week meetings with a group of parents of handicapped children to teach them how to help their child. We agreed to take part and that the organisers should come to meet us and Will to study his development. They then hoped at intervals to monitor his development both before, during and after we had participated in the project.

Two women came one summer morning. They tested his reactions, his physical development and his human responsiveness. The thing that took me by surprise was my own reaction to their visit. I found myself being very eager to "show off" everything I knew Will could do. It revealed to me that far from having an unconcerned un-competitive attitude about how he was I was most concerned not only that he was doing well but that he should be seen to be doing well. Equally interesting and, I found, touching was that at the time we had a friend staying who had during his stay grown close and involved with Will. He too was present that morning and he too was equally concerned that Will should be seen to be doing the best he knew Will could do.

There was no doubt that considering Will's handicaps

he was coming along very well if unevenly. His physical mobility development was slow, but his other responses were not much behind that of a normal child. He had learnt to grasp and play with things, watch things and smile. He was obviously very aware and responsive to everything going on around him, particularly responsive to people's faces. From early on, almost from the moment he could focus, his eyes went to the human face. This was true throughout his life. Almost every photo of him depicts him either looking at the person who is holding him or looking at the person who is photographing him. Even when he was feeding he would often be at my breast looking up at my face. As he developed, his human responsiveness and warmth were very evident. They were also very endearing. We, the doting parents, were not the only people to come under this particular form of his charm.

Medically, Will remained throughout that period in the capable and sympathetic hands of the Home Care Unit. Dr Z visited every week and gave him a check-up, weighing him, listening to his heart and lungs, and discussing with me his feeding and general development. As we got to know each other better we would discuss Will's handicap. She brought me a medical article to read and told me of other facilities, like speech therapy, which she would be able to arrange for Will when he was older. One of the questions she always asked was whether Will was ever breathless. In fact Ed noticed and commented on his breathlessness first, I soon noticed it and it became more evident the more he tried to move about.

During one of Dr Z's visits, after she had given Will his weekly check-up, she sat down on the bed which was in the room and I sat down too. She then told me she could hear a heart murmur. She put it very gently, said she didn't know the extent of the heart trouble but that she was convinced that she could hear a murmur. Compounded with his breathlessness the symptoms were worrying. Obviously she had made sure she could hear something before saying anything, especially since the consultant had quite firmly said that he could hear nothing. She explained what we already knew, that congenital heart defects were one of the major physical problems of Down's Syndrome children. Although we knew the fact, having read it in almost every piece of literature we had read about Down's Syndrome babies, we did not really take it in or believe that Will might have that too. We had glibly told people that the infant mortality rate of Down's Syndrome children had been greatly reduced by two major medical advances, antibiotics and heart surgery. Somehow we believed that Will came within our glib generalisation. Dr Z said that for the time being it was not necessary to take any action about his heart but just to watch it carefully and to be very careful that he didn't catch a cold.

I cannot remember our precise reactions to the fact that he had a murmur. We were worried and one of the ways my worry manifested itself was to make me even less willing to leave him with anyone except someone whom I felt was absolutely responsible and capable. We discussed it and Ed kept reassuring me that many people lived perfectly normal lives with heart murmurs – that there was a first division footballer with one.

I heard on the radio one day, the day of the year given to mentally handicapped children, a poem written by the father of a Down's Syndrome child which had died from a heart defect. It shook my confidence but it was built up again by stories we heard of other children who lived with heart defects or who had survived heart surgery. Life continued much the same except that anyone with any infection was barred from the house. People with colds in particular were told to keep away. We took Dr Z's warning very seriously that if Will caught a cold, with a heart murmur he could be "in trouble". There was one panic. He had a bit of a sniffle but it didn't develop into anything more serious. The warm summer was under way and life with our little baby was surprisingly rewarding.

7. THE FUTURE

I can't remember the precise date but sometime during the summer I received a telephone call from a producer at the BBC. He said that he had heard that I had a handicapped baby, that he has been thinking of making a documentary on the subject based on one family, and could he come round to discuss it with me. I was non-committal but agreed. I do remember very vividly his arrival. For the first ten minutes I let him make the normal BBC film maker's approach to people they are trying to interest in co-operating in a programme. It was unfair of me but I couldn't resist it. I was experiencing being at the receiving end of a process in which before I had always been at the giving end. So finally I came clean and admitted that not only had I made (directed) documentary films but had also on occasion made them for the BBC. He realised then that if we were seriously to discuss a possible film it would have to be as two professionals. Though of course in the last analysis, he would be the one making the film and I would be the one the film was to be about.

Obviously before any further move was made Ed would have to be involved. Further discussions did take place involving Ed and we reached a basic agreement on the structure of a film that we all accepted. Both Ed and I felt strongly that we did not want to be involved in a film which would be just a personal profile of two people with their handicapped baby. If we were to be involved we wanted it to be a film at the end of which people would not just think of our particular situation but that of handicapped children in general. The basic structure which the producer suggested and which we agreed to was one based loosely on, or rather inspired by, Humphrey Jenning's *A Diary for Timothy*. It would take this small baby Will as the central person and look at, through us his parents, the kind of life we could expect for our child. It was to me a challenging structure for it would have enabled me both to explore what the actual situation is for handicapped children and adults in our society and also to make my comments about it.

The prospect of the film set me thinking, reading and asking questions about the position of handicapped children, the facilities available to them and their parents and of what the future might hold for a handicapped adult. Much that I found out was deeply depressing.

But whilst the position of handicapped people or their relatives is appalling, one is continually overwhelmed, despite all this, by the humour, courage and fortitude of many people in that situation. Our first experience of that and our first insight into the future for Will came when he was about four months old. A friend suggested that if we wanted to talk to some other parents of a Down's Syndrome child (one who was now adolescent) she could arrange for us to meet her friends and their child. We hesistantly accepted an invitation to dinner with her and her friend Mrs B. Driving to the dinner, Ed and I both felt apprehensive. We both resisted the idea that because we had a handicapped child, we too were handicapped and that we were being drawn into a world of the handicapped. Within five minutes of our arrival our fears were completely dispelled. We quickly realised that the B's were a normal family, conducting a normal life but with a handicapped child as part of it. For us both it was a very positive experience, in a number of ways.

Mrs B had two other children whom she was sure, and I did not doubt her, had been enriched rather than deprived because they had grown up with a handicapped sister. She worked, entertained, went on holidays and led a normal life. Her husband had obviously been a great help and support throughout and both talked of their situation and of their daughter with humour and humanity. I left the dinner feeling that for me, as a woman, life could and would go on and that I need not be totally submerged into the small enclosed world of handicap.

For both of us the evening was also rewarding in other ways. Before going we had both been nervous about meeting Anna, their daughter, for we both realised that it would be our first glimpse into the likely future for Will. The first impression was a shock. At the physical level Anna looked clearly Down's Syndrome with the immediately recognisable features and small stature. But like all abnormalities of looks, particularly not very marked ones and Anna's were not that marked, they soon recede on acquaintance as the individual's personality takes over. Ed in fact was more worried by her physical appearance than I was and later he commented to me that he was glad Will was a boy because "looks" still matter much more for a girl in our society than for a boy. Quite quickly Anna's personality began to impress itself on us. Her speech was limited but it was quite obvious that she had developed a sophisticated form of non-verbal communication. We both felt that probably because she had learnt to communicate so well with few words neither she nor others had bothered to press for better speech which she might have been capable of. She could do all the basic things about the house such as making tea, dressing, cleaning, and so on, and we were told that she was a great "entertainer", mimickry being her forte. But above all there was no doubt that she was a warm, friendly outgoing person with great emotional sensitivity. Anna gave us a lot in our brief meeting in terms of confirming our belief in a positive future for Will even though we would have to come to terms with its limitations.

Instinctively Ed and I had thought that a handicapped child should be brought up in the family if at all possible and Anna was proof of it. Thinking about the B family in trying to clarify my thoughts for a possible film I began to question from what beliefs and conditions society's attitude towards the mentally handicapped had been moulded.

I did not research the history of attitudes in any thorough way but from the little I gleaned it seemed clear that prior to the nineteenth century, apart from a few "loony bins", most mentally handicapped children and adults remained in the community. There was nowhere else for them to be. Mocked maybe, they undoubtedly had, like all members of the community, to contribute to it to the best of their ability. A Down's Syndrome child that survived into adulthood, probably a rare phenomenon, would have been given some simple task to do as a matter of economic necessity. The fact that handicapped people were in the community meant that the rigid distinction we have between normality and abnormality could not have been sustained. It also must have meant that people had to accept a very wide spectrum of human behaviour and abilities within the community.

The removal of mentally handicapped people from society came with the industrial revolution. Along with the introduction of the division of labour came the division of the population into productive and non-productive. Society was divided into children, workers, women and old people and further into the normal and the abnormal, the latter being non-productive adults who were "removed" from society. Of course the wealthy could, where they wished, buy their way out of those divisions but for most industrialisation meant the imposition of divisions onto their life and work.

The nineteenth century brought increasing institutionalisation of the mentally handicapped, society providing minimal care so that people did not actually die but not much else. Nineteenth century liberalism also nurtured the charitable instincts of some of the wealthy and the mentally handicapped provided an outlet for these. Amongst those motivated by christianity there was also the belief that God created the mentally handicapped so that normal people could gain salvation through good works towards those less fortunate than themselves. Sadly that attitude is still evident in some of the charitable organisations established then and still existent today. Whilst handicapped people require help it needs to be based on a recognition that they have a right to that help.

Liberalism and the relative wealth of Britain has meant that, although the care of the mentally handicapped leaves much to be desired and in some cases is still horrific, they are only "removed" from society, not from life. Soon after Will was born a friend lent me a bound copy of *The Times* for July/September 1945. Whilst looking through it for articles about women workers I read reports that the Allies had found in Germany concentration and extermination camps for the mentally handicapped. It was a sharp reminder that fascism was not just based on racism but that it was also an extreme form of capitalism in which any non-productive worker was redundant. It was also a very chilling realisation that my child, under fascist rule, would have met such a fate.

Although the care of the mentally handicapped has improved enormously in Britain this century, it is still based on the removal of the handicapped from society into special schools, institutions and workplaces. This has led to a great deal of fear and ignorance. Most people prefer not to be disturbed and for threats to be kept at a safe distance. Some have always challenged that attitude, but recently there has been a wider change, mainly amongst those directly concerned with the mentally handicapped; it is now widely believed that mentally handicapped people should remain in society at every stage of their life.

The struggle to begin to integrate them must necessarily begin with the family. In recent years families have been encouraged to keep their handicapped child and not to put them into care. This move has not only been supported and led by those working in the field including parents but has also been backed by the government, at least in theory. In many cases now great social and emotional pressure is put on the parents to keep their child at home on the basis that it is best for the child. Given the right conditions I believe that to be true. However, the theory conveniently fits in with government economic policies of cutbacks in public expenditure. It is much cheaper to have a child supported by its own family than kept at the state's expense. The main burden thus falls almost invariably on the mother. The back-up services, the practical support for the policy (a policy also endorsed by local authorities) are noticeable by their absence. As I began to look into what help and support we might get I found that we could expect very little.

In theory, help should be available from the outset. On leaving hospital with a new born handicapped child, by law one's local authority should be informed and the parents should be visited at home by a social worker. We were never visited or contacted by a social worker or anyone else from the local authority apart from the routine post-natal visit from the health visitor. From those that I have talked to our experience was common. Given that most parents are not visited by any professional person one wonders how they find out what services are available except by accident or through their own tenacity and determination. Since it is a situation that many people are embarrassed about, many are undoubtedly inhibited about looking for help and information.

Apart from a GP, the first professional advice and especially the first professional advice on the child's development may well come only when the child is "assessed" for schooling – help that comes five years too late. By that time many opportunities for helping both child and parents have been missed. One of the most important services that should be provided for all children and particularly handicapped children is that of nursery schooling. However, since the provision for child care in day nurseries and nursery education is generally so abysmal and currently being cut back only a minority of children have access to it. In our case we did find that the local state day nursery took a small quota of handicapped children and that we might at a later date possibly get a place in it for Will. There would have been many advantages to that but also disadvantages. Because there are so few day nursery places available they are reserved, as in most state day nurseries, for a quota of handicapped children, disadvantaged children referred by a social worker or children of one parent families. The benefits to all concerned would be much greater if there were enough day nursery places and nursery school places for all children so that in each there could be a social mix. Such a mix is important for all children but particularly important for Down's Syndrome children who even more than others learn by imitation. For this reason alone it is very important, if the child is to integrate, that the behaviour around them which they are imitating is predominantly "normal".

The other great importance of the provision of child care facilities for all ages is to enable the parents – and particularly the mother – to lead some kind of life away from the child. Even if the mother does not wish to work the strain and tension of caring full time for a handicapped child can be physically and mentally draining. A break is what parents need and is what most parents find so hard to get. Very little is provided at any stage. Besides the great shortage of child care provision for the under fives there is an even greater lack of provision of child care facilities for the over fives. One or two local authorities provide short-stay homes and short-stay foster homes where a child can go for a weekend or a week whilst the parents are away for a holiday or just having a break at home. It is a service every local authority should provide for all people caring for handicapped children or relatives. Some authorities and organisations also organise holidays for handicapped children but again far too few.

It is not surprising that many families either break up or end up by putting their child, reluctantly, into care. With so little support provided the burden on the family is very great. We were warned by various people, including my GP who suggested that Ed and I should get married, as if that would help, that we might well at some stage have to face making a decision between our relationship and our child. It was also pointed out to us that the rate of marital breakdown in families with a handicapped child was very high. The decision to choose between my relationship and my child was one I could not imagine but I could understand the kind of pressures which lead people into having to make it. For many it is a heart breaking one and those who choose to put their child into care often find that they then have to live with an almost intolerable guilt. As it happened we were never put to the test of coping with disruptive behaviour, of being permanently tied – the seemingly endless struggle which forces people into that decision. But I am sure that far fewer people would be forced into it if the burden and the pressures on them were alleviated by the provision of real support services and if the attitude towards the mentally handicapped were more enlightened.

When I began to enquire about the kind of education we could expect for Will, it was with horror that I found out what the situation was. At five, handicapped children are "assessed" and, on the basis of that assessment, a decision is made on the education the child should have. At best an assessment is made by observing the child over a long period of time, but sometimes a decision is made by a person who does not know the child, on the basis of one short period of assessment in a strange environment. A few Down's Syndrome children are accepted into ordinary primary schools but the vast majority go to special schools for the handicapped. There was some improvement in 1978, when the Warnock Committee recommended that handicapped children should be educated with other children. However, the principle of integration had not been established in 1975, and even now there are relatively few experiments.

Evidence from a variety of sources has shown that the potential of Down's Syndrome children is much greater than had ever been assumed. Obviously that potential can be realised only if the child is given the right stimulation and environment. In this instance the United States is far in advance of Britain not only in theory but also in practice. The state of Massachusetts pioneered the practical application of the theory that handicapped children should be integrated into the normal state school system. Early experiments were given legal backing in 1974 by a state law, the Bartley Daly Act. This Act marked a great breakthrough. It stopped the categorisation of children into normal, sub-normal and severely sub-normal and replaced it with the concept of children with special needs. By doing so it removed the stigma of the former categories – categories we still have in Britain. Children with special needs are defined by the Act as anyone who "because of difficulties arising from intellectual, sensory, emotional or physical factors, or other specific learning disabilities, is unable to progress in a normal school programme". Such a definition covers a very wide range of children. The Act lays down that children with special needs are to be catered for within the normal school system and not taken out of it. The onus is now on the schools to provide the special services and teaching which the children need. Whilst it has taken time to re-organise the school system the benefits from the change of policy have already been felt. One example reported in a *New Society* article on the working of the Act shows how different life could be for all handicapped children if the Massachusetts example were followed:

"In Wayland School, a junior high school of 300 children, there are eight children who would have been described as 'trainable retarded' (British term 'educationally sub-normal') before the act. There is no special class and it is not always possible to pick these children out. All children with special needs, like other children, move around the school for classes. Linda, a 14 year old mongol girl, attends normal classes in science, physical education, social studies, art and music, and receives some special help in maths and English. 'Special needs can be short-term', one teacher told me. 'Everyone is liable to have some problem or other at some time. It is not just the slowest children who use the resource centre.'"

Linda reads at an eleven year old level and is a sociable child. In Britain, as in some states in America, she would automatically be sent to a special school for the severely subnormal because of her diagnosis of mongolism. Under the Act she not only has the opportunity to learn and play with normal children, but will also move to a high school to continue her education until she is 21, if her parents wish. So far in Britain there have been only one or two experiments at such integration at the nursery and primary school level and it seems that legislation to enforce integration is a long way off.

As I found out what the situation was actually like for handicapped children and what it could be, were there the political will to change it, I found myself becoming increasingly angry. The thought that my child might be shunted off into a school for the handicapped appalled me. It increased my resolve that I would both do everything I could to help Will reach a level of development which would make him acceptable in a normal school, at least at the primary school level, and it also increased my resolve to fight for the wider change needed so that all children could be integrated with the exception of a very few very severely handicapped. Quite quickly I realised, like so many other parents of handicapped children must have, that I would have to struggle for the right of my child to have a meaningful place in society. Later I learnt that some even have to fight for the right to a chance of life for their child. Handicapped people are second class citizens. As someone who does not believe in second class citizens, whether women, or workers, or migrant workers, or old age pensioners I was certainly not going to accept such a status for my child.

Fortunately at all stages of my search for information there were always some positive examples. Mrs B had been one of them. Finding out about the Bartley Daly Act in Massachusetts was another. There were several more. Before Will left St A's hospital I had a long chat with the sister and she recounted to me the story of a Down's Syndrome man she had known who had worked in a hospital laboratory. She remembered him well and described him in great detail. I remembered it because it was the first example I had heard of a Down's Syndrome adult doing a normal job. Others told us of people they knew with Down's Syndrome children at normal schools. Someone lent me an extraordinary, bizarre book called *The World of Nigel Hunt*. It was written by a Down's Syndrome boy. I saw a Down's Syndrome man in the tube obviously going about his normal business. They and many more were examples of what could be achieved and they gave me great hope.

Examples of Down's Syndrome adults integrating into society were particularly important for me. The fear which I had had five minutes after the news was broken to me about Will as to what would happen to him when he grew up remained ever present.

I feared for what would happen to him if we died before him; I feared for how I would cope with having an adult dependent on me for the rest of my life; I feared for how society would treat him as an adult. Whilst people are usually sympathetic towards a handicapped child, sympathy is absent in most people's treatment of handicapped adults. The options for a handicapped adult who cannot live an independent life are bleak and equally bleak are the options for the responsible relatives. Either Will would have to go into full time residential care in a home or a hospital or he would continue to live with and be dependent on us. The likelihood was, as the life expectancy of those with Down's Syndrome is considerably shorter than that for normal people, that he would predecease us, but we still worried about what would happen if we died first.

The thought that he might, at any stage of his life, have to go into full time residential care appalled me. Full time care even at its best would mean he would be removed from the normal world in which I believed he had a rightful place. At worst it would mean he might end up in a mental hospital where in some cases the level of care and conditions are appalling and inhumane. The other option, that he would be dependent on us in his adult life, was also hard to face. Although limited work is provided in "sheltered workshops" the environment and the work in most is unstimulating even to those of a low level of ability and the pay is based on charity, not a living wage.

Given the main options it was not surprising that I found every exception that I heard of so encouraging. Obviously the most encouraging were of those few Down's Syndrome adults leading independent lives. Such a future was almost more than I dared to hope for for Will. Given the present attitude towards the handicapped one of the best alternatives was a few self-supporting communities for the handicapped which I heard about. In them the handicapped can lead dignified lives, working to support themselves, needing only minimal help and living in "family" units.

In my searches there was one question I didn't, or dared not ask because I was frightened of the reply. It had saddened me to think that Will might grow up denied the possibility of a loving sexual relationship with another person. To talk about the sexual desires and needs of a mentally handicapped adult is to touch upon a very sensitive subject – almost a taboo. It arouses a very deep-rooted fear of the mentally handicapped; one that has been fed largely on myths of their almost demon-like, uncontrollable sexual urges. This is combined with a belief that the mentally abnormal will reproduce themselves and their abnormalities. There is undoubtedly a long long way to go before we understand, recognise and help the mentally handicapped in terms of their sexual needs and desires. The question I dared not ask was that if Will fathered a child would it have Down's Syndrome? Much later I found out the answer. If it was with a normal woman the chances would be 50/50 – if with a woman with Down's Syndrome it would be Down's Syndrome. The question of fatherhood aside, I did hope very deep down that Will could be loved by another person, yet the reality was that it was very unlikely. That hurt and saddened me.

I merely thought about all these things. In the course

of the summer it emerged that Will's heart trouble was something much more serious than a slight murmur. It was agreed that the film should wait until after the investigations into his heart had been completed.

8. THE CHOICE

One summer's morning in July I woke up and Will had a cold. I phoned Dr Z and she came round that morning. Having listened to him and confirmed that he did have a cold she prescribed some antibiotics and something else called digitalis which she explained to me was a heart stimulant. Normally someone in the Home Care Unit, either Dr Z herself or the sister, brought me any necessary drugs which had been made up in the hospital pharmacy so that I did not have to traipse round chemists finding the right drugs in the form and strength suitable for such a tiny baby. On this occasion Dr Z left the prescription with me as I had told her that I planned to go down to my parents for the weekend. My parents lived only an hour and a half's drive away and I thought that I would collect the prescription when I arrived there. En route I stopped at some friends briefly and there it was evident that Will was in distress. He was having difficulty in breathing, his nose was very blocked and because of that he was having difficulty sucking. My friend's husband offered to go to collect Will's prescription. He was away a long time having gone to several chemists before he could find one who had what was required. I gave Will his first dose and continued to my parents' home.

Soon after arriving I began to get quite frightened. Will was breathing with difficulty. At one point my mother had him sitting on her knee and he began to go blue. For some reason she laid him on his back. I shouted at her "sit him up, sit him up". She did so and he returned to his normal colour. That night was a long and frightening one. I stayed up with him almost all night. He slept fitfully and I tried to keep him, whilst sleeping, with his head slightly raised, but he would keep sliding down flat onto his back, get into breathing difficulties, begin to go blue and would have to be rescued. In the morning he was slightly better and during the day he gradually improved. Dr Z had not explained that the digitalis needed about twenty four hours to take real effect. Once the pressure eased I remember sitting crying, tired and frightened. I phoned Ed and asked him to come down both for his support but also to accompany me on the drive home. The prospect of driving on my own, with Will at the back in his carrycot and being unable to see him worried me. Ed came down on the Sunday and we returned to London. Although my parents were of great help in looking after me I felt I wanted to be in London with Dr Z on call.

On the Monday morning Dr Z called again and pronounced him much improved. She was obviously pleased to see him better and was very sympathetic about the fright I had had. I did not call Dr Z again that week as Will, although a little below normal, appeared to be on the mend. Quite by coincidence at the end of that week I had to take him for a routine check-up with the consultant at the children's hospital. I told Ed it was not necessary for him to take time off work to come with me this time and that I could cope.

After what seemed to be the inevitable wait I went into the consultant's room with Will. He asked me how Will was and I explained that he had had a cold, had been put on digitalis and antibiotics but that he seemed to have recovered. He was eating and sleeping normally again. I was quite confident. The consultant looked at Will, listened to his heart and then turned to me and said "We'll have to admit him, he's in a state of heart failure." No further explanation was given. I was shown into a neighbouring room and handed over to a nurse who was to arrange for his admission. The shock was terrible. For a long time I was left on my own sitting in the bare room, holding Will and feeling dazed. After finding out that it would be some time before Will was actually admitted I phoned Ed and in tears asked him to come to the hospital explaining briefly why. Ed came. We hung about, waited, were shunted around. During the long wait it seemed to me an extraordinarily casual way for a hospital to be behaving towards a tiny baby with heart failure, a condition which sounded to me fairly critical.

When he was finally admitted it was done by a young American doctor who quickly realised our dazed, frightened and mystified state and began to explain what was meant by "heart failure" and also what they would try to do in hospital. They hoped to arrest the heart failure by finding the right level of stimulant for his heart and diuretics for his kidneys. The doctor asked us if there were any questions we wanted to ask. Once again we could ask little about Will's condition as we did not know what questions to ask but I did ask if it would be possible, as I was still breast feeding Will, for me to stay in the hospital. He arranged for me to sleep in a spare nurse's room and then left telling us where, when and how we could contact him in case there were any further problems or questions we wanted to ask. I went home, packed a few things and moved into the hospital. Will had a little room of his own with glass walls and I spent most of his waking time with him. When he slept, I ate, walked about, met Ed in the evenings but did little else. Although I had taken books with me I couldn't concentrate enough to read. On the second day the American doctor said that he would arrange for Will to go and see a consultant cardiologist. The next day, accompanied by a student nurse, I took Will to the heart hospital. There were the usual waits and delays before we went in to see the consultant, Mr X. He read the letter which we had brought with us, asked me a few questions and then called in two of his colleagues. The three of them proceeded to discuss Will in language way above my head. Finally Mr X apologised for not explaining what they were talking about but he didn't go on to explain anything except to say that they would want Will to come into the heart hospital for a few days in the near future so that they could do some investigations into the exact nature of his heart problem. We had planned to go up to Scotland for two weeks' holiday and I asked if it would be safe for me to take him that far away and was told that it would be. Mr X explained that if Will started deteriorating he would, most likely, do so slowly. Almost ominously he said "Yes, I think you should have your holiday." Looking back on his remark I am sure he was thinking, "take your holiday, for you're going to need all the strength you can muster for what is to come".

Waiting for the taxi to take us back to the children's hospital I managed to persuade the student nurse to break the rules and join me for a drink. It was a warm day and we sat, me with Will on my knee, outside the pub and had a modest glass of lager each. Back at the children's hospital the American doctor carefully explained about the investigation they would do on Will. He also explained to me what symptoms we should look out for if Will's heart did begin to be under strain again. Dr Z also dropped in on me at the children's hospital and we had a quick cup of tea and a chat together. The next day Will was allowed home. This time I took him home much less confident. My fears were beginning to grow.

The day after, Ed left for Scotland. He had to teach for two weeks at a summer school, a contractual obligation of his job. I had a bad two weeks at home. The weather was warm and oppressive. It seemed to intensify my mood.

Those two weeks were the one period when I really felt trapped with my child. I also felt resentful that I had to take so much of the responsibility for Will, not just in terms of time and care but also, since I was always in the front line with him in coping with doctors, in terms of the emotional strain. What I really wanted was that the burden should, like the joys, be equally shared. Illogically in my resentful mood I thought that if ever Ed and I broke up my claim to Will would be undeniable. I was very glad when those two weeks came to an end.

We had arranged that I should travel up to Scotland with Will by train and that we would meet in the Highlands at the house where we were to stay. Two friends took me and Will to the station and put us on the train. I felt like royalty, being escorted to the first class sleeper I had treated myself and Will to. I was met in Pitlochry by an old friend whose house we were to stay in. Ed arrived a day later having picked up a hired car which we thought we might need in case of an emergency.

We had a glorious ten days in the Highlands. The weather was beautiful, in fact so hot I swam in the Loch on several occasions. I talked to Ed about my feelings of resentment and in just talking about them they melted away. The little cottage we were staying in was on the south side of Loch Tummel with beautiful views in every direction. Our friends were good company and they had a little girl who was absolutely fascinated by Will, particularly by his being breast fed, and on the last day she sat down beside me, picked up her doll and announced that her doll was also going to have some "titty for tea". The holiday was a perfect break. A break in which we relaxed, enjoyed Will, enjoyed each other, ate bowlfuls of wild raspberries and drank rare malt whiskys.

Fairly soon after returning to London in early September I received a letter from the heart hospital giving me a date on which to take Will in. The investigation they wanted to carry out was what is called a cardiac catheter; where they put a fine "tube" into a vein and ease it up into the heart. By doing that, they can find out the existence, nature and size of any hole (or holes) in the heart chambers. During the course of the investigation, done under anaesthetic, they can also find out other important information.

Once again I moved into hospital with Will. This time he had a whole room to himself and I had a little bed in it, which I could put up at night and fold away in the day time. Once again I was thrown into the state, induced by hospitals, where the rest of the world recedes and you become consumed by the immediate problem. Fortunately it was a relatively short visit, five days, and it went without complication. Before I left they gave me the first results. Unfortunately Ed was not there at the time, as he came to the hospital in the evening and the consultant's round was in the morning. The consultant, Mr X, told me quite briefly that Will had a defect of the heart, in lay language, a hole. I understood the word "hole" but little else. The news was hard to assimilate and confronted with about ten people in the room, the complement that seems to make up a "consultant's round" I felt too inhibited to ask any questions. Much to my relief the senior registrar, Mr Y, with whom I had had several long conversations already, turned to me as they were leaving the room and said "Don't worry if you don't understand. I'll come back later and explain." He did come back and when he returned he had a large chart in his hand. It was a diagram of the heart. On it he showed me the type of hole Will had, a large one right in the middle called an atrial/ventricle canal. He explained that they could already tell us this much but that we would have to wait for a while, until they had analysed other data before they could know the full picture. When the analysis had been done, Dr Y said, we would be called to the hospital. He also said that they would then be able to discuss with us what the options would be.

Soon after my return home with Will Dr Z came to see me. She had been in direct contact with the hospital and wanted to make sure everything had been clearly explained to me. I sometimes wondered how I would cope without her visits. I grew to rely on her, knowing that she was always there to explain things, to talk to, to be consulted. Over the months we had built up a strong friendship, never overt or explicit, but a friendship we both felt. During our conversations, nearly always brief because Dr Z was always in a hurry, her work load being far too heavy, we had slowly found out about each other, about each other's work, culture, attitudes and had found we shared much. From the outset I had never felt with her a doctor (superior)-patient (inferior) relationship and from talking to one or two other parents I met who knew her I found out that they felt the same.

Back at home life went on as normally as it could. Ed and I started attending the weekly group sessions run by the Institute of Psychiatry for parents of handicapped children. My parents kindly made a commitment that one or both of them would come up once a week to baby-sit so that we could attend the classes. One thing we quickly realised at the class was that Will's handicap was far less severe than that of the children of most of the other parents in the group. We did at least have rewards – feedback. He laughed and smiled. He responded very positively, making you aware that you were with a quite distinctly individual human being. It was also clear that his development in terms of social reactions, manual dexterity and things like hand/eye co-ordination were good. But his physical development was quite definitely retarded. It was obvious he had a second handicap, a physical handicap, his heart. He was beginning to want to crawl and was trying to sit up but he had very little energy. He was quickly tired and became breathless from very little physical exertion. At that stage it was hard to work out what was due to physical handicap and what to mental handicap. Much less hard to work out was our reaction to his problems. Faced with his heart the problem about his mental handicap receded.

Ed and I both went with Will to see Mr X at the heart hospital for our arranged appointment. In fact when we arrived we initially talked to the senior registrar Dr Y. He repeated what he had said to me before about the nature and size of Will's hole but he said that in the light of the other information they had acquired they thought that his condition was operable. He stressed that it was a major defect but that a few such operations had been attempted and some had been successful. Each operation of that magnitude was slightly different so that it was hard to make a prediction about the success or otherwise of the operation. He also explained that whilst they could get a pretty clear idea of the size of the hole from the cardiac catheter, until they actually "opened him up" they wouldn't know what complications there would be. Since the hole was so large it would be a case of patching it, not as satisfactory as having a normal heart but, if the operation was successful, it would mean that whilst his heart would never be as strong as an unpatched one he would be able to lead a physically fairly normal life. Dr Y also described what the probable future would be for Will if he did not have an operation. His life expectancy would be short. He could not predict how short, whether months or years, for that would depend very much on other factors, but it would be short, always prey to a fatal cold or infection. His heart would increasingly incapacitate him, stunting his growth and restricting severely and increasingly his physical mobility. Dr Y recommended we choose the operation, saying that that was what he would advise for a normal child and adding that in Will's case, the combination of a mental handicap with a physical one would make for a very bleak life. We asked only one question, "what were the odds on the operation, what were the chances of it being successful?" The answer we got was not the one we wanted but it was, I think, an honest one. He answered by saying that it was a relatively new operation, one which a few years back they would not even have attempted. They were having an increasing success rate and were learning and becoming more proficient at it all the time. However, he did stress that an operation of that size and complexity on such a tiny baby who might present other complications because of his Down's Syndrome would obviously be a great risk.

Given the choice of the possibility of life or a slow death for Will both Ed and I chose immediately and instinctively the possibility of life – the operation. We told Dr Y there and then of our decision and assured him we did not need time to think about it. Dr Y said that before we finally committed ourselves we should discuss it with the consultant, Mr X. He went to ask Mr X to join us which he did without delay. Dr Y explained briefly to him that he had told us what the situation was and that we would like to opt for the operation. Mr X then offered us a different perspective, one which shattered me. Up to this point we had been talking with Dr Y about our child as any parent talks about a child that they love and cherish. There was an implicit assumption, shared by him, that parents want their child to live. Suddenly we were being offered a different option, of letting our child die. We found ourselves sitting there being told by Mr X that if we didn't want to choose the operation, that if, because of our child's handicap, we wanted them to leave our child (inevitably to die) they would respect our decision. Fortunately Dr Y knowing us, and me in particular, and probably sensing our shock, quickly interrupted and said that in his discussion with us he was sure the operation was what we wanted and that they should go forward on that basis. It was agreed that we should – and so soon as there was an operating date available.

We left the hospital shattered. We had just made a life or death choice for Will – one in which, in fact, we felt we had no choice. But much more shattering was the very stark way in which it had been brought home to us that our child was a second class human being in some people's eyes. It was most hurtful to realise that because he was a Down's Syndrome child leaving him to die was an option. Some months later, fortunately months after Will had had his operation, I read an article in the *Guardian* in which this attitude was clearly revealed. The article was an interview with a Dr Elliott Shinebourne, a consultant paediatric cardiologist, who talked about the great work that was being done and had been done at the children's heart unit. His main message was that we in Britain are as advanced as anywhere else in the world in children's heart surgery. That was a point I would not dispute but I did and still do dispute which children he feels their work is designed to benefit. At the end of the article he commented:

"We are here, though, to help children who can go on to live normal lives. I do not personally believe that we should do all we possibly can for a child that is maybe brain damaged or mongol, though I do respond to parents' wishes on this. I would not want to help keep a life if that child was going to be severely retarded. One of the things we have to contend with is whether with our fancy surgery we are keeping alive babies whom nature would have let die."

Carol Dix who conducted the interview sharply wrote "For most parents involved the question is not so confusing. They know they want to be able to defeat nature." I would have liked to have added my own comments and questions to him. What do you mean by nature? Is nature only to take its way with some children and not others? Is not the whole heart unit a superb example of our attempt to defeat nature? Mr Shinebourne, do you think you have the right to arbitrate on which part of nature should be defeated and which part should be left to take its way?

By circumstance we found we had been directly caught up, and involved, in the large and difficult problem of what level of health care should be provided by society and for whom. Born in 1944 and brought up in the welfare state I had assumed that any medical care that there was should be available to those who needed it. That belief had been slowly but quite firmly eroded. The erosion started slowly but gathered speed during the past few years with added momentum given by the government cutbacks in public expenditure. It is now clearly the case that the level of health care varies greatly from area to area, that there are many long waiting lists, that there are many people who do not get the care they need and that we are not all equal in the eyes of the National Health Service. Due to shortages of facilities decisions are being made all the time as to who should have what and when. The decisions are not just about minor "luxury" medical needs, they are about life and death – kidney machines, heart surgery, expensive drugs such as those needed for haemophiliacs.

If we are to accept the reality that decisions must be made as to what society can provide, or rather wishes to provide, in terms of health care, then the question is who should make those decisions. It is clear we cannot, unless there is a radical change in our economic system, provide the unlimited care those of us who were brought up in the first flush of the welfare state were led to expect. We therefore have to make decisions. No government to date has had the courage to admit publicly its priorities in terms of health care, even less has any had the courage to say we cannot afford XY and Z so they will not be provided. But in practice that is what is happening. By refusing to give money to one hospital or cutting the budget for another, or in refusing to train staff for another or put money into research government cuts reduce the level of health care and in doing so also establishes its priorities.

The lack of courage on the part of governments and health authorities to make public policy statements about their priorities in health care mean that much of the onus of decision-making falls on the doctors. It is doctors who decide which patient gets the kidney machine, and doctors are not free from their own particular prejudices and beliefs. It is not only unfair to patients that doctors should be deciding who gets what; it is also unfair on the doctor. It frequently puts the doctor in an invidious position. If there were no pressure on places for children's heart surgery, doctors would not have to decide between children. Also if society was prepared to pay the money to provide the help, education and stimulation that Down's Syndrome children require Dr Shinebourne and many more like him would not, I am sure quite so glibly wish to refuse to offer them a chance of life and leave them to "nature".

9. DEATH

Having chosen the operation all we could do was wait, wait for a letter to come from the hospital with the date. Dr Z visited me regularly. Her first visit was the day after we had been to the heart hospital to make our decision about the operation. She phoned me and asked if she could call that morning. When she arrived it was clear that she had been in touch with the hospital and had been informed of the situation and of our decision. Normally when she arrived we would go straight to see Will. This time she said she would just like to talk to me.

We sat on the sofa. She began talking. She had brought a book with her which had a section in it on the particular operation Will was to have and she gave it to me to read. It was her way of trying to tell me that Will's chances of surviving the operation were very slight. I respected her greatly for feeling she must tell me, knowing how hard it was for her to do so.

Finally the letter arrived. We were to take Will in on 17 November, the operation being planned for the 19th. I had been both fearing and looking forward to the letter. I both wanted to know the date and dreaded it. With a date I knew what time we had. Time which is possibly finite takes on an entirely new dimension. You live completely in it for you don't know if there is going to be any more. That time has to be all time.

Once we knew the date and told other people, it was clear they sensed that time might be finite. It was a great emotional strain. I remember my father visiting me and I knew he was in tears as he left. My mother came and the parting was, I knew for her, heart rending.

During that period I used to have one very simple day dream which kept recurring. I imagined myself sitting on a large sandy beach in the sunshine and that Will would come running up to me and laughing tumble into my lap. It was a dream but, as do many daydreams, it reflected my hopes. My hopes were strong. I just kept hoping.

For Will that period was uneventful. The last entry in my diary of his week by week development reads:

"*Weight*? Looking v. fat and chubby. Weaned except for a suck at breakfast. Loves bottle – eats from spoon well except still doesn't like savouries. On three meals a day with afternoon tea of milk.

Mobility Still not sitting on his own – though sits with minimal help. Once sat bolt upright in his pram for about 5 mins. When leaning back pulls himself forward. Still loves standing – pushes with legs and pulls with arms to get up into standing position. Can do it with minimal help. Not crawling – does crawling motion with knees but can't co-ordinate arms and legs. Seems much more motivated to standing than to crawling. Rolls over tummy to back frequently – strong arms.

Much more sociable smiles a lot – blows raspberries, tries out noises like shouts and squeaks but apart from 'B' has made no other identifiable speech noises. V. wary of strangers – sometimes cries with them. Takes him some time to check them out and then relaxes with them.

Very aware of his surroundings – watches everything and listens to different sounds. Interested in the mirror. Great watcher of everything including television, also great listener and continues to obviously love music.

Playful – feels everything and puts everything in his mouth but paper still his favourite. Fairly clumsy at getting hold of things but manages."

On the morning of 17 November we drove to the hospital. Ed had taken time off work. We knew we had to be together. Will was admitted and then subjected to the gamut of tests which had to be done before the operation. We stayed with him most of the time. For the first two nights I slept at the hospital where there was accommodation for mothers only, but a room had been reserved for us in a house opposite the hospital which was owned by the League of Friends and made available to both parents over the critical days of the actual operation. It was reassuring to know that we would be able to be alone in privacy together in the immediate vicinity of the hospital during the critical time.

Tuesday 18 November was a long day. There were more tests. My mother arrived unexpectedly to visit us three. There was also the grand consultant's round. Before taking Will to the hospital, when he blew raspberries we would jokingly say, "now you mustn't do that to the consultant – it's not very polite." Will took no notice. As usual the consultant, Mr X, swept into the room on his round followed by a bevy of white coated workers and one in blue, a staff nurse. Dr Y, who was one of the bevy, was asked to give the information on Will's case. He started, "This is William . . . he's . . ." and continued with a long spiel about him. With perfect timing and just as he finished, Will, who was being held by Ed, blew a large defiant raspberry at them all. Only Dr Y smiled and called Will "a poppet" and I saw the nurse repressing a smile.

I got up very early on Wednesday morning. The last food Will was allowed was at six. It had been agreed that I should be allowed to breast feed him then but it was stressed that he must not have anything else. I sat there and let him suck and suck. By that point I had little milk left as he had been weaned off all other meals and it was his last. I had meant that he should have been fully weaned before he went to the hospital but I couldn't bring myself to stop that last feed. Sitting there I wanted Will to take any strength from me that he could. As at the beginning it was, I felt, the one thing I could give him.

Ed arrived early at the hospital. We breakfasted together in the canteen but neither of us could eat. The rest of the time we spent with Will. He was washed and gowned for his operation and given a pre-med. We just took it in turns to hold him. At about one o'clock they arrived to take him to the operating theatre. He was still awake. They wheeled him away in his cot. He disappeared down the corridor lying on his tummy looking up at us. We turned away choking back the tears.

We had decided that we would leave the hospital and not return until the first possible time there might be any news. So we walked around, tried eating, attempted to distract ourselves and ended up by returning to the hospital at four o'clock, an hour before we could expect to hear anything. We waited and at five enquired if there was any news. There wasn't any. At six, as instructed, we asked again. This time Dr Y was there and he said he would go and see what was happening. He was away for what seemed like a long time. When he came back he told us that things had been bad, that at one stage they didn't think they'd "get him off the table" but that things were improving and they were hopeful. We were told to go to the room that had been reserved for us and that they would phone us there. It was another two hours before they phoned to say that Will was, at last, being moved from the operating theatre to the intensive care unit and that in about an hour's time we could see him. Before going to see him I phoned my parents to say that Will was still alive. They said that they would drive up to London and spend the night in our house so that they would be near in case we needed them.

At about nine we were allowed into the intensive care unit. It was an awesome experience. Will was lying on a small high table. His whole torso was swathed in bandages. There were electrical gadgets all round – drips, blood, monitors. Ed counted seventeen tubes or wires going to and from, in and out of his body. There was even a tiny thermometer bandaged between his toes. The thing that impressed me most was the respirator. I called it the breathing machine. It thumped the air into his tiny body. We saw him briefly. It was hard to relate to him in that situation, unconscious, swathed by technology. You could only hold his hand, which I did. We were asked if we could return at about eleven when he would be well established in the intensive care unit. At eleven the prospect looked good. The doctor was optimistic. Will's heart beat and blood pressure had stabilised. We went to bed with hope.

Early the following morning when we arrived at the unit the surgeon was already there. He was looking worried. He told us that he was concerned about Will and could we go away and come back a bit later. An hour later we returned and were kept waiting outside. We could just see in enough to realise the doctor's concern was with Will at that time and not with any of the other five or six children who were in the unit. The nurse who was monitoring Will (each child in the unit had a nurse permanently with them) told the doctor that Will's toe temperature was 33.0 C. Ed worked that out as 91 F. His calculation might not have been quite accurate but it was obvious Will's toe temperature was low.

Finally we were allowed in to see Will on condition that our visit was brief. It was. I just held his hand a moment. We said we would return to our room and they assured us that they would phone if there was any change. We waited. The phone went but it was for someone else. Then the phone went again. Ed answered. By Ed's reaction I knew the news was bad. Will had had a cardiac arrest. The prospect was not good. They said they would phone again.

Soon after the phone rang again, again Ed answered. This time I saw him crumple, controlling his choking just long enough to hear the news. He didn't need to tell me. I knew Will was dead.

We both wept.

Sometime later the hospital phoned to ask if we wanted to see Will.

I was hesitant but Ed was sure that he did. We both went. It was the final reality, a reality so devastatingly real it seemed unreal. But it is that final reality, that final memory that is imprinted on me irradicably. That is death.

10. GRIEF

I was totally unprepared for Will's death. Although I had known he might die and had imagined his death, all my imaginings of what it would be like, how I would cope, what I would do had not prepared me at all. The shock was total. I had believed he would live. I believed and hoped until the last minute.

After seeing Will we talked to Dr Y. We sat in a tiny office and he said how sorry he was and we believed him. Dr Y explained that complications had arisen during the operation. When they opened up Will they found not only the hole which they knew about, in itself a formidable task to mend, but also that both valves were badly defective. The surgeon had had to repair them too and it had taken a long time. A critical factor in open heart surgery is the length of time the operation takes. They have to freeze the heart for the operation and the longer it is frozen the harder it is to get it to function properly again. That, Dr Y thought, had probably been the most important factor in the failure. But finally Will had died of renal failure too. He talked about whether they should have started dialysis, and said that they didn't normally do so at that stage so they hadn't and perhaps that had been a mistake. In fact they didn't really know what had gone wrong but it was probably a combination of factors. We were asked to sign a form allowing them to do a post mortem so that they might understand better what had gone wrong, which might help them in future. We agreed and Ed signed.

Dr Y then said that if, after the post mortem, we wished to talk to them further about the cause of Will's death we could. Always, before, I had wanted to know at every stage exactly what had happened, what was happening and what might happen. It had often been hard to extract the information, except from Dr Z who always gave it to the best of her ability, but I had always sought it in one way or another. Now I was no longer interested. Will was dead and there were no more questions I wanted to ask about his life.

The only question I remember asking what "What do we do now?" Dr Y did not know how to reply. I meant the question in the general sense and in a particular sense. I realised that he could not answer in the first sense but only in the second so I quickly rephrased the question to "I mean, what do we do now, I mean there are things to organise and things. . . ." "I think you should just go home and later it can be sorted out." So Ed and I walked out of the hospital dazed, shocked and fragile and the only help offered to us was to "just go home". I felt we were an embarrassment to them. Not just to Dr Y but to the whole system. Despite the fact that it must be a situation with which they have to deal quite frequently they had no training, no personnel, no organisation to deal with it. They are there to fight for life and when that life ends their role in relation to that life and those involved ends.

We did however have another support system, our families and friends. My parents had come to the hospital that morning feeling they might be needed. They arrived shortly after Will died. My father got there first having come on ahead whilst my mother parked the car. I opened the door to him. He was smiling and looking confident so before he could say anything I stuttered "he's dead" and was immediately taken, like a child, into his arms and held. My mother arrived soon after and my father broke the news to her. When she came in the room she didn't say anything but just went and embraced me and then Ed.

It was, given the public nature of hospitals, a great privilege that we could face our grief in private. The provision of such facilities by the League of Friends was something we deeply appreciated. It is a facility which should be made available to all hospitals and I think is particularly important for men. The pressure on British men not to give way to showing grief in public is very great. The privacy enabled Ed to break without inhibition. Breaking is the first step in enabling one to grieve and then to come to terms with one's grief.

Thanks to my parents we did not walk out of the hospital feeling alone. We went home and my parents followed after they had packed our things, talked to the hospital about the formalities and collected Will's things.

The first stage of grief is total – the mind and body are totally consumed in one emotion. The mental shock is a physical shock. I felt cold, very cold and kept adding layers of clothing. I felt sick as though I had been kicked in the stomach and couldn't eat. My mother, hoping to entice me to eat, sent my father out to buy a little smoked salmon one of my favourite foods. In the evening I ate a little of it but could not swallow any bread. I cannot eat smoked salmon now without remembering.

Both of us drank what was probably quite a lot of whisky, but we did not feel any effect, our grief seeming to consume the alcohol. People had talked about heart ache, but it was only then I realised it is a physical sensation.

On that first day we phoned one or two people to tell them. I wanted people to know and know quickly. I also wanted to forestall phone calls from people asking us how the operation had gone. The first people we phoned were those who were close, very close. Those whom we knew would feel the pain. Those phone calls revealed the terrible limitations of the phone and of words. The message was simple, the response straight and simple but the words so difficult to say by both parties. We got enormous strength from people's responses. As soon as C heard, an old and close friend, she came round. There was little concrete she could say or do but her presence was strength.

Ed and I stayed at home that night, retiring to our bedroom. We needed to be alone and my parents respected that need. The following day we agreed to go to my parent's house for a day or two. It was to put some space between us and the terrible emptiness of our house. Before going we had to make arrangements for the funeral. My father made the initial inquiries but Ed had to face the decisions about details. Reluctantly he accepted that Will would be cremated. Much to our relief my parents also dealt with registering the death and getting the death certificate, saving us the ordeal. Before leaving London the date time and place of the cremation had been arranged and we asked C to phone our friends both to tell them the news and tell them of the arrangements for the cremation.

After lunch we left. C stayed to help my mother clear up our house. I was grateful, for it would have been a lonely, painful job for my mother to do on her own. It was a job too I was grateful I did not have to face. I could not bring myself to go into Will's room.

At my parent's home in Kent my father arranged for me to see their doctor. I still had milk in my breasts, not so much that there was any physical discomfort but enough to be a painful reminder of the living bond. Considerately I was allowed to see the doctor just before his surgery opened so that I did not have to wait in the waiting room. Between sobs and tears I explained my problem. He refused to prescribe anything explaining that the drugs that had been formerly used to "dry up" milk were now thought unsafe.

As he was explaining it to me I remembered women at the hospital being told exactly the same thing when their milk came through after the birth of their child. He further added that the shock would probably dry my milk up quickly. I accepted his refusal to prescribe anything but I felt he had little understanding of my anguish. He did however give me some valium which I had not asked for, I had not even intimated that I felt the need for any such "treatment". I took the prescription and left. I knew I didn't want valium but I didn't argue. I had the prescription made up at the chemist's, but the pills were left untaken, except on the day of the cremation.

I did not take the valium because I felt that whilst it might be a help in the short term, in the long term it would probably be a hindrance. Both Ed and I felt that grief was something we had to face, to feel, to confront and hopefully some day come to terms with. We felt it had a natural course, one which we did not understand but one which we felt had to work its way out. Since neither of us had experienced the death of someone so close our feelings about how we should face grief were quite instinctive. Taking valium to me seemed a way of either delaying or evading what had to be faced. I also felt that to repress my grief by one means or another would probably in the long run make it much harder to come to terms with.

When I left the doctor once again I was left with the impression that he too, like most of his colleagues, was unable to cope with such a situation. Admittedly he was a doctor I had never seen before and one whom I was not likely to see again but I doubt if things would have been much different with any other. He, like so many others would have done, prescribed valium because that is their frame of reference. Such "treatment" is also quick and easy. It is easy because it is in line with the way doctors have been trained and is in line with the body/mind duality that appears to be a premise of medicine as learnt and practised in Britain. Many patients have also come to expect and to accept a prescription from a doctor believing that such "treatment" can cure or cope with any mental or physical problem.

Perhaps my expectations of doctors, ones I share with many other people, are too high. However those expectations have been created partially by the medical profession themselves. It would seem that if they are to meet them the medical profession needs to radically change its training, its practice and its attitudes or it should admit that its practitioners have neither the time, training nor inclination to deal with such situations and that the gap should be filled by other trained people.

Besides somehow coping with the fact that we were alive and Will was dead we spent much of the six days between Will's death and the cremation thinking about what form the ceremony should take. As neither of us has any religious beliefs we naturally did not consider any form of religious service. Having ruled that out we were then faced with what to do and what to say. The absence of any ritual surrounding death leaves the bereaved in a vacuum. Rituals do provide a framework of behaviour for people in unfamiliar situations. They also provide ways and forms in which other people can relate to the bereaved when they too do not know how to behave or what to say. But rituals can only work when they are meaningful to those they concern. And since the religious one was meaningless to us, we had to create our own way of mourning Will's death.

Both of us felt very strongly that we wanted to make a statement about his life, about our feelings about his life and by implication our feelings about his death. We suspected that many people thought that because he was a Down's Syndrome child, because he was "different", our feelings might be different. We also suspected that many people would be thinking "it's really for the best". Later we didn't even have to suspect that that was what people were thinking, some told us so. The measure of his life was that those people who had known him well grieved with us, we felt, with no reservation. He had changed us and them.

Besides wanting to make a statement we knew we wanted the whole ceremony to be simple; anything else would have been totally out of place with his life. Finally we chose a piece of Wordsworth which I asked a friend to read. We also asked my friend C to say a few words about him. She based what she said on a few things Ed wrote, something my father wrote, but put it in her own words and added her own comment.

This is what C said:

"Sarah and Ed have asked me to say a few words about Will. We'll follow with a few moments of silence and then Kathy will read some lines from Wordsworth.

I'd like to start with some lines from Robert Lowell which say:

> *'And love lives on and hath the power to bless
> When they who loved are hidden in the graves.'*

In his short life Will had a special capacity for happiness which brought great happiness to Sarah and Ed and to all who knew him. He was a handicapped child, a little mongol baby, and he was no less a human being, in fact to Sarah and Ed and all of us, it made him more special. No one who knew him failed to respond to the warmth of his smile and to feel that he was a fellow creature. As Sarah's father said, he had a smile that came right out to meet you with a real feeling of fellowship and of communion that enriched the lives of Sarah and Ed and all who met him. Will indeed had the power to bless and his blessing will I'm sure, live on.

Children like him increase our knowledge of what it is

to be human. Will helped to broaden our understanding and enrich our lives.

Will brought out in Sarah and Ed a capacity for profound love, caring and understanding which affected me, and I'm sure, everyone who knows them, very deeply. The short period of his life was both a difficult and an enriching time. Their response, their power to love, gave me personally a sense of the magnificence of human achievement.

The knowledge of that love will survive with us always."

The extract from Wordsworth was from his *Ode on Intimations of Immortality from Recollections of Early Childhood*:

> *What though the radiance which was once so bright*
> *Be now for ever taken from my sight,*
> *Though nothing can bring back the hour*
> *Of splendour in the grass, of glory in the flower;*
> *We will grieve not, rather find*
> *Strength in what remains behind;*
> *In the primal sympathy*
> *Which having been must ever be;*
> *In the soothing thoughts that spring*
> *Out of human suffering;*
> *In the faith that looks through death,*
> *In years that bring the philosophic mind. . . .*
>
> *Thanks to the human heart by which we live,*
> *Thanks to its tenderness, its joys, and fears,*
> *To me the meanest flower that blows can give*
> *Thoughts that do often lie too deep for tears.*

As planned the ceremony was simple. Afterwards everyone came back to our house for drinks, food and tea. It was nice to be surrounded and cushioned by warmth and support. In the following weeks we received many letters, cards, telegrams and messages (one a single orchid) and bizarre presents that touched us deeply from my sister's children who had spontaneously decided to give Ed and me something. Dr Z, who had been away during the week of Will's death, called to offer her sympathy as did the sister from the Home Care unit.

We drew strength from all the sympathy and support people gave us. The fact that people contacted us in one way or another was important. After such an event has happened you cannot meet people again as if nothing has happened. Some way that change has to be communicated and the fact that people contacted us meant that when you next saw them or got in touch we knew that they knew so that the "ice" had been broken. But before we faced that we decided we had to put some time and space between us – our lives that had to be lived – and his death.

11. HIDING THE WOUND

I remember thinking before Will died, "I will have to go a long way away if he dies." That was what in fact we did. We were lucky in that we had the money to do that. Many people do not. Having decided we wanted to go somewhere far away our choice was governed by wanting sunshine and by flight dates. We wanted to leave immediately (within a day or two at the most) of the cremation. Having studied the travel brochures, much to the surprise of the travel agent we walked in on the Monday and asked to book for a two week holiday in the Seychelles leaving on the Friday. Being late November there was no problem booking so on the Friday we left for our most expensive "holiday" ever.

It was a strange, strained two weeks in many ways, the place being so contrary to our mood. Still unspoilt, the Seychelles as viewed by the tourist are tropical paradise islands. There are coral reefs, empty sandy beaches, warm clear sea, coconut palms, exotic fruits and flowers, rare birds and amazing underwater life.

Most of our holiday Ed and I existed in our own world of grief. We didn't socialise at all but we found the very relaxed atmosphere of the hotel and the islands in general very soothing. Although we didn't socialise we did decide to do things. Having gone so far we thought we should see as much as possible. It was good for us to have the stimulation of things that were rare, beautiful and exotic. Always too there was the sun and the sea. We could sleep and build up some strength. Doing things made me realise just how physically drained and exhausted I was.

There were times when the grief would just well up and overflow. Sitting on the beach I remembered my day dream and wept. Watching a baby sitting playing in a pool of water made me have to turn my back and hide my tears. The pain was never far from the surface.

Back in London we had to face the re-entry. Ed went back to work. A friend of mine had arranged for me to do a short job as a researcher immediately after Christmas. Until I started that job I made myself busy, but I can't remember what I did except to make a dress and a cloak. We joined in the Christmas festivities but without much enthusiasm. By the time I started to work I thought that I had gathered enough strength to cope with it. At one level I did but at another I found it a great strain. Most of the people I had to work with did not know what I had just been through. I was faced with the problem: do you tell strangers, or do you pretend that nothing is wrong? I ended up by telling those I shared an office with and I expect the word went round. The producer who had planned to do a film about Will was at that time working in the same building and I found it a relief talking to him.

During that period of not knowing whether I wanted to tell people or not, I almost longed to wear a black armband just as an outside symbol of my inner fragility. I wanted people to know without having to tell them. When people don't know you fear the comment, the joke, the association which you know will strike a chord in you when you are unprepared, a chord of which you cannot control the vibrations. Memories suddenly forced on me, that took me unawares, would make me break. There was a particular Fats Domino song which I used to dance to with Will in my arms. I would dance to the rhythm and at the chorus "You left me reeling and rocking" I would begin to rock him quite violently and he would always burst into laughter. One day suddenly I heard it on the radio. I could not control my reaction. It was the same with many other things. On the other hand, emotionally prepared, I could remember many things about Will in calm.

There were other aspects about grief that I was unprepared for, like the length of time one grieves and the different stages one goes through. One stage I found particularly difficult was when "normal" life had resumed or, at least, when to the outside world my normal life had resumed. I was working, going out and being involved in a variety of things. At home our life had returned to normal. The normality of a couple without children. We closed our bedroom door at night. We slept in in the morning. The house was tidy, the kind of tidiness of no children. A photo of Will in the front room was the one reminder to those who visited us that things had been different. For those who went upstairs there was another reminder, Will's room tidied, untouched and unused. But the surface belied my emotional state. Although I had reached a stage of being able to do other things Will was always in my mind. I wanted to talk about him but most people evaded the subject. The one or two people who did let me talk or who openly asked questions about how I was feeling were of enormous help. Ed found the same. We also both found we needed to talk to other people, not to each other. Although we had developed a great closeness and sensitivity to each others' emotional states we found it difficult to talk to each other as we found it too upsetting. We both needed other people who were not emotionally involved.

As that stage of grief dragged on I began seriously to think I needed help, outside, possibly professional, help. I felt trapped in my grief. I had difficulty sleeping and when I did sleep I had vivid nightmares about death. During the day

I couldn't liberate my mind from thinking about Will. But the problem was where to look for help. My brief encounters with the medical profession didn't give me much confidence, particularly since I rejected their type of help, drugs. They would also, I knew advise me to have another baby quickly, which was, I thought, just another way of evading the problem. I considered going to a phsycotherapist or a psychoanalyst but rejected that too on the basis that I did not feel abnormal. What I was going through seemed a normal human emotion, that of grief, and analysis seemed inappropriate. What I felt I needed was the help and guidance of someone who knew about grief, who knew the stages, whom I could talk to and who could advise me. Unfortunately I felt I could not approach the only two people I knew who had experienced the death of their child. At that point I did not know that an organisation called Compassionate Friends had been started by parents who had lost a child themselves, and whose purpose was to help other parents in the same situation. Had I known about them I would have contacted them. Failing to find anyone I felt I could go to for help meant that I had to help myself.

My form of self-help was work. I threw myself into it. After a brief period of research I returned to my book. There was a lot left to do. I managed to settle down to it. It was work that was interesting and that I enjoyed. I could become and became absorbed. That was followed by other projects – a film, radio programmes, all equally absorbing. I also returned to active involvement in my trade union.

The self-help therapy did work in a way. It did enable me to move out of that stage of grief in which I had felt trapped. It also helped me to re-establish my own sense of independence and identity. As I built myself up I began to realise the many sided way Will's life and death had affected me.

At one level, like most women returning to the world

of work having been in the world of babies, children and the home I felt much less self-confident particularly at first. But my lack of confidence was exacerbated by the fact that so many assumptions, so many things to do with normality, to do with life, to do with relationships, had been questioned and challenged for me during the preceeding year that I felt unsure of my base. In the process of returning to work my base did become redefined. It was not fundamentally different from what it had been before; rather my former base was re-inforced. For instance the work I first did after his death was work I knew I would not particularly like but I had taken it because I thought it would be good for me to get out of the house. I was grateful for the offer and it was nice to earn some money again. In fact its effect was to drive me back home to the work which I was committed to and believed in. Having to do research for a programme in which a serious subject was treated superficially, almost whimsically, was even more unacceptable to me after the experience of Will than it had been before.

As I faced up to the world again I realised that I felt stronger because I knew myself better. Having had to face things which I had never faced before made me know much better my own strengths and weaknesses, my own possibilities and limitations. It made me both much more tolerant and intolerant of myself and of others. Tolerant of people's weaknesses, handicaps and limitations; intolerant of people who don't use, or worse, abuse their knowledge and privilege. The experience of Will had also made my priorities much clearer. Once again it was not a radical change. After having questioned my value system I found I was to re-affirm it but this time with much greater surety based on a better understanding.

It was an intense year for me. I had to do everything intensely, even my "leisure" pursuits had concentration about them. Behind everything I did there was a driving force – the fear of stopping. I felt I had to keep running because to stop was to think and to think was to remember. I hadn't come to terms with Will's death. My grief remained close to the surface. My life was largely one of evasion, my actions motivated by reaction to Will's death. I chose my main form of doing, "work", for a variety of reasons. It was helpful to me not just because I found it interesting and absorbing. It was a refuge too. The world of work is well protected from the world of babies, children and motherhood. The separation of society into self-contained worlds, particularly the separation between work and children and the home is one I deplore, a separation that is a product of an industrialised, male-dominated society. Because of the respective roles of men and women it is a separation which most men have not questioned but many women have. A working mother cannot help but be aware that her life cannot be so neatly and conveniently divided. Fortunately more and more people, both men and women, are becoming aware of those divisions and are questioning them but radical change seems still a long way off. Much as I deplore it, I took advantage of it for that brief period in my life. As a childless woman I could take refuge in that separation. Obviously I could not evade totally the world of children, babies and motherhood and there were moments when it was painfully brought to my notice but it is surprising just how much you can. Not so surprising though for many men since it is an evasion which they manage for most of their lives.

12. A NEW LIFE

Very soon after Will died I knew I wanted another baby. Any attempts to conceive, however, were temporarily inhibited by the fact that I was still using the coil. A more important inhibiting factor was that the obstetrician had advised me to have an x-ray of my cervix before getting pregnant again. This would ascertain whether I had a cervical weakness which might mean that a second child would also be born prematurely or whether Will's prematurity had been caused by his abnormality. The fear that something might go wrong in a second pregnancy made me refrain from trying to conceive until after the x-ray. But there were delays. First I had to have my coil removed. Then I had to wait and my waiting was extended by the fact that the machine at the hospital was out of action. It all took months. Finally I got the medical go-ahead to conceive but in the meantime Ed had been offered a job in the States for the first five months of 1977. If I had conceived then, the baby would have arrived whilst he was away, so we delayed trying until the autumn. Late autumn 1977 I conceived again.

I had been very impatient with all the delays. The final delay caused me to feel that Ed did not really understand my need to have another baby. He felt I did not understand his need for the job in the States. But once I had conceived we forgot our mutual misunderstandings. They were taken over by our pleasure. In fact all the delays were for the good although I wasn't aware of it at the time. If I had conceived immediately after Will's death I don't know that I would have taken the physical strain. I was weak and exhausted. It was only months later when I began to feel stronger again that I realised just how drained I had been. It was important too that Ed went to the States; it would give him a stimulating break from his work routine.

There was however a much more important reason why I am glad I did not conceive again immediately. After Will died I did not want another baby, a new unique individual, I wanted Will back. I wanted to re-create an identikit of him. In fact I think the conventional advice given to people by doctors and lay people alike that after the death of one child they should "have another as quickly as possible" is irresponsible. It is advice that considers the parents but not the child-to-be. Another child should start life as a new individual and not under pressure to replace the dead child. That advice implies that you can *replace* a dead child, that you can replace people. But people are not replaceable as human beings. Of course immediately after Will's death I did not question my desire to replace him. The delay of a year before conceiving again made me, at least, aware of the problem, but my awareness didn't teach me how to cope with it.

The first three months of my second pregnancy were awful. I suffered from morning sickness and from nausea all day. Like some frightful torture, the terrible taste in my mouth never left me and all that time I didn't know whether I would be going through with the pregnancy or not. After the diagnosis of Will's Down's Syndrome my obstetrician had told me that if I got pregnant again he would offer to perform an amniocentesis so that at least the possibility of Down's Syndrome could be averted in a second pregnancy. An amniocentesis is a test in which a little of the amniotic fluid from the womb is extracted with a hypodermic needle. Cells of the foetus can usually be found in the fluid and these can be cultured in a laboratory. A cultured cell is then subjected to a chromosome analysis. From that the doctors can then tell whether there is any chromosomal abnormality in the foetus (the most common being Down's Syndrome where there are 47 chromosomes, more precisely the 21st pair having an extra one, in each cell instead of the normal 46). From the chromosome analysis they can also tell the sex of the foetus. The amniocentesis was offered to me on the assumption that if anything were found to be abnormal I would agree to a termination of my pregnancy. In fact it was spelt out to me that they perform the test on the understanding that a termination would be carried out if anything was wrong.

The issue did not seem that simple to me. Firstly there are risks to the test although those are being diminished all the time, as it is being performed more frequently and obstetricians are becoming more experienced at doing it. The precision and safety of the test has also been increased by the use of ultra sound. The person who convinced me that the test's medical risks were very small compared to the risks of abnormality was Dr Z. We had discussed it at an earlier stage and although she had advised me to have the test I remained unsure. She convinced me when she herself got pregnant again and wrote to tell me that she had had an amniocentesis.

There was another much more difficult problem for me related to the test, a psyhological one. If everything was found to be all right then it would be easy but if anything was wrong and in particular if the foetus presented a Down's Syndrome chromosome structure what would I do? It was a problem few understood. Like the obstetricians, most people assumed that I would want to terminate the pregnancy. It was an assumption founded on their attitudes towards me and the handicapped; attitudes which varied from, at one extreme, those who assumed sympathetically that I would not want another handicapped child because of all the problems it would cause, and those, at the other extreme, who believe we should use the developments of medical science to ensure the reproduction only of "normal" people. From people's assumptions I realised they would regard it as irresponsible of me to knowingly bring another handicapped child into the world. If I did it would have been my decision and would then have to be my responsibility. I should not expect others to offer the support and help which they had offered to us and Will. On the other hand I knew that if I made the decision to terminate the pregnancy of a Down's Syndrome foetus I would be betraying Will. I would feel as though I was betraying not only him but all that I had fought for, for him and by implication for others like him – his right to a chance of life, to an education, to a place in society, to human dignity.

It was a difficult problem which I knew I could partially evade by not having the test. Finally after much heart searching we did decide that I should have it before Ed went to the States and that if anything were wrong I would terminate my pregnancy. I resolved to abide by our decision. The actual amniocentesis was carried out quickly and easily. I had a nervous twenty-four hours wondering if it would provoke a miscarriage followed by almost three weeks of nerve-wracking waiting for the result. Unfortunately they cannot perform the amniocentesis until the 16th – 18th week of pregnancy and then it takes at least two weeks to get a result. If anything is wrong one is faced with the prospect of a late termination, always medically complicated and psychologically traumatic. (When a pregnancy is ended for medical reasons it is called a "termination", when it is ended for social reasons it is more emotively called an "abortion".)

Throughout my pregnancy but particularly during

that waiting period at St A's, whose ante-natal clinic I attended, they were very considerate of me, of my body and of my obvious fears. It was the same hospital I attended for Will's birth. The sister who ran the clinic was helpful and understanding. When I requested that I should see the same doctor at each visit and not just anyone on duty, she readily agreed and wrote the doctor's name in large letters on my file. She also wrote and underlined in red my previous history so that others would not make the same mistake as she had done when first interviewing me by saying, "This is your second pregnancy, how old's your first?" Despite her attempts to warn people, most did not notice and time and time again I was asked the same question or a similar question by nurses and students. Each time I visited the clinic hoping the results of the test had come through and was disappointed she was sympathetic, helpful and somehow always found the time to give one special consideration.

Finally the result did come. I had to wait whilst they sent to the laboratory for the photo of the chromosome structure. Whilst the doctor was telling me it was all normal my eyes frantically scoured it to see if there was an extra chromosome. To my relief they were all arranged neatly in 23 pairs. I burst into tears. The relief was overwhelming. The only other thing I could take in was that the "it" was a "she". We were going to have a girl. Seeing my reaction and relief must have been quite an experience for the laboratory technician who had brought over the photo. She stayed in the room whilst the doctor told me and it must have been rewarding for her to see for once positive results of her work.

Having got the result I immediately rushed home and phoned Ed in the States. Down the phone I spluttered "It's alright, it's a girl." He was clearly delighted to be woken up to that news. I then rushed around re-organising my flight to the States which had had to be cancelled because of the delays in obtaining the results of the test. I then made lots of other excited phone calls spluttering out the same good news to friends and relatives who were all also obviously pleased to hear that "it" was alright but not quite so sure how to react to the fact I said I knew "it" was a "she".

The rest of my pregnancy wasn't easy but it was a lot easier than the first three months had been. My five week visit to the States was a diversion in mid-pregnancy, but for the rest I never managed to really get involved enough in my work to divert me from my fears. Although some had been eliminated by the amniocentesis I continued to worry about all the other things that could go wrong. I had to spend the seventh month in hospital resting, a precaution against Jessie arriving prematurely. By that point she was named and we felt we were just waiting for her to be born so that we could be introduced. It didn't worry me at all that I knew the sex of my foetus. I did not feel that it would detract from the excitement of the actual birth or take, as some people argued, the mystery away. There was also, after having seen the double XX on her chromosome structure, no doubt in my mind that "it" was a "she". Other people were not so sure. I remember a phone call to a woman I didn't know, to whom I had to explain that I couldn't do something because I was expecting a baby and *she* was due in July. The woman immediately said, "you mean you *hope* it's a she". I explained I didn't hope, I knew. She then commented that obviously I was such an ardent feminist that I was willing my foetus to be female.

The only disadvantage I felt to knowing the sex of my unborn child was that she immediately became more personalised. That would only be a problem, I thought, if for some reason I miscarried or had a still-birth. In that eventuality I am sure I would have felt even more that I had lost a particular person.

The hardest thing for me about going into hospital for

that month was having to re-tread steps, steps which I knew would bring back memories. I had hoped to evade confronting such memories until Jessie was actually born. I thought I would then have the strength to face them. In a panic the day before I had to go in I phoned my mother to ask if she could accompany me to the hospital as Ed was still in the States. Since it is a small maternity unit I dreaded that they might even put me in a bed in the same ward that I had been in after I had had Will. That did not happen but I was given a bed in the ward next door. I could not help but see each day the bed in the ward on which I had sat when I had been told that Will was a mongol. Likewise I could not evade passing that single room in which Will and I had struggled to establish breast feeding. As upsetting was the fact I couldn't evade the world of babies and motherhood. It was all around me and for a few days, because the other wards were full, a mother with a new born baby was moved into our ward that was normally reserved for ante-natal patients only. I buried myself in books, the radio and in knitting, consoling myself with the belief that it would be all right once Jessie was born. I expected that miraculously at her birth, I would suddenly be able to stop running and begin to really re-build.

Ed returned from the States just before I came out of hospital so the last month of my pregnancy I spent at home with him. Jessie arrived at the predicted time. My labour was quick, easy and uncomplicated. I hadn't bothered doing any exercises to prepare myself as all I cared about was that she came out healthy and normal. A mid-wife actually delivered me but I was surrounded by other people. Ed was there. This time he was much more relaxed and able to enjoy it all much more. Two doctors that had cared for me during my pregnancy were also there. They came in just before the moment of birth to watch "Baby Boston" being born. Unfortunately they arrived at the only bad moment in my labour. The second stage happened so quickly no one had the time to give me an episiotomy so instead of being neatly cut, the pain of the cut being numbed by a local anesthetic, I tore. The terrible pain of the tearing was quickly overtaken by the appearance of Jessie's head followed by the wonderful moment when her whole body was finally delivered. Straightaway she was laid down on my tummy. She wriggled and cried and seemed even at the moment of birth, vibrant. She looked normal. She was alive. I put her to the breast and she sucked. Effortlessly she knew what to do. I was amazed. Ed and I took turns in holding her and drinking the cups of tea that they had brought for us.

Although the mid-wife said she looked "normal" and Ed and I could see nothing wrong with her I didn't feel entirely confident that nothing was wrong. I wanted her to be checked by a paediatrician. She was born at mid-day and by the following morning she still had not been checked, although I had asked the sister about it. Eavesdropping on a conversation between the woman in the next bed and a doctor I realised that he must be a paediatrician. I went up to him as soon as their conversation was over and asked if he would check my baby as soon as possible. Briefly I explained about Will as a way of saying I was not just a neurotic mother but did have reasonable grounds for my worries. The doctor looked at me and said, "Of course, Mrs Boston," (as a matter of convention they call all mothers married or otherwise Mrs in maternity hospitals) "I remember you and Will." As he said that I realised who he was, behind the large bushy beard he had grown since I last saw him. He was the registrar who had cared for Will during his first six weeks of life in intensive care and who had supported me throughout the struggle to breast feed him. It was nice having him check Jessie, which he did there and then. There was that ease of relationship which comes from each understanding the other because of what you have experienced together. I could feel my heart race and my hands go clammy as he waggled her feet, moved her legs and arms, looked at her head and listened to her heart and breathing. Apart from mild jaundice he could find absolutely nothing wrong with her.

For the rest of my brief stay in hospital (less than three days) I was high – high from relief, ecstasy and from the energy gained from the life force of birth. Everyone shared my delight. Doctors, friends and relatives, the sisters from the ante-natal clinic and from the intensive care unit all visited me and were visibly pleased. On the third day Ed came to pick us up to take us home. We were a happy, proud threesome which left the hospital.

I was totally unprepared for the emotional struggle that was to hit me when I got home. I had assumed everything would be all right once Jessie was born. It didn't work out like that. Although I was determined that Jessie should be a new start and that I should not try to make her a replacement, it was much harder than I had expected. Part of my attempt to give her a new start was giving away all of Will's personal things. We sent to the heart hospital all of his clothes and toys. I bought everything new for Jessie. To have dressed Jessie in Will's clothes would have made me look at Jessie and think of him. But despite all my efforts, physical and mental, to fight that reaction I didn't succeed. I remember holding Jessie in my arms and weeping for Will.

To hold a baby again, to change its nappies, to feed it and play with it just made me re-live doing all those things with Will. It made me confront all I had been evading since his death. No one had warned me that such feelings are common following the birth of a second child when the first has died. I felt guilty that I was mourning Will when I had Jessie and because of my guilt I could not talk about the fact that I was going through a second period of mourning for which I had been totally unprepared. I felt even more guilty that there were times when I resented Jessie because she was, in those first few months, so difficult and demanding. Her brother, I would think, never demanded anything and yet here she was demanding all the time.

Another problem which both Ed and I thought we might have was that we would be neurotically overprotective of Jessie. In fact it was a problem I found much less difficult to cope with and it was one other people were much more understanding about. Fortunately, for the first year of Jessie's life she was remarkably healthy, which made it easier. Although we were, and still are, undoubtedly more protective of Jessie than many parents are of their children I think we manage most of the time to behave and react in a reasonably balanced way. Sometimes we lose that balance. The first time she was ill we both found particularly difficult. She had quite a severe attack of bronchitis and just as she was beginning to get better she started vomiting which frightened both of us. I remember Ed just bursting into tears and I knew the tears were a sudden welling up to the surface of memories and fears. From time to time if Jessie is ill or has a fall I get a tight sick feeling in the pit of my stomach, but mostly I feel I can lead a normal life and let her lead a normal life.

My problem in relating to Jessie and in coming to terms with the fact she was not Will were solved more by Jessie than by me. As she developed and grew, asserting herself as a very definite individual, I compared her less and less to Will and began to relate to her as Jessie. I mourned less and less for Will and became more and more involved with Jessie. I had loved her from birth, but I had to develop a love for her as Jessie not as an image of someone I had lost.

Jessie is now for me a person totally in her own right. She has not replaced Will but she has placed herself very positively in our lives. She is a little person who delights, amazes, exasperates and moves me. She is a source of great happiness to Ed and me.

Developing my relationship with Jessie meant coming to terms with the death of Will and with my grief. The sheer force of her individuality helped me to do that. With her help, with Ed's love and support and with the support of so many other friends and relatives, particularly my parents, I now feel I have come through.

I remember Will mostly in calm but sometimes even now memories jog me and I break. I still want to talk about him not so much because I any longer have a need but because to be silent about him is to deny his existence. Time however has not stopped me feeling bitter and hurt when people say his death was "for the best". But time and events have stopped me running away from his death. Now I run, because like Dr Sassall interviewed by John Berger in *A Fortunate Man*, "Whenever I am reminded of death . . . I think of my own and this makes me try to work harder." Such running is an affirmation, not an evasion, of life and in my case an affirmation of the preciousness of time and love. That is Will's legacy.

HOW TO FIND OUT MORE

Information, or lack of it, was one of the ever-present problems I faced throughout the period covered by this book. Ignorance, for me, was not bliss. Ignorance was fear and continual worrying. Looking back on it I think of how easily some of those worries and fears could have been averted by a little information given at the right time. Like most people catapulted into similar situations I was in every sense a "lay person", and as such I was doubly handicapped: by the fact that I knew nothing, and that I was unaware of what I did not know. It was only slowly that I did find out most of the questions I wanted to ask and usually, one way or another, the answers.

Often I wondered how parents in less privileged positions than myself, and with far more limited access to sources of information, found out anything at all. Yet the giving of information, often vital to the well-being of both the parents and handicapped child, could be easy. Less easy, but equally necessary, is the making available of advice and experienced understanding to bereaved parents. These services should be an integral part of the National Health Service, but in my experience they are either not available or split between a plethora of people with different areas of skill and knowledge, so that ignorant parents are likely to slip through the whole system, with their problems ignored.

Almost all parents I have talked to, heard or read about

in similar situations have also found that information is rarely given but has to be sought. And they have found that what is given is usually inadequate. All too frequently the "givers" take the attitude that the "receivers" can't "take more", or "understand more" or even have the right to "know more".

For those who do want to "know more" I thought it appropriate to give a resumé of some of the sources of information and advice which I found helpful. It is *not* a comprehensive list of organisations and literature on the subject, but rather a personalised list of the groups, people, books and so on which helped me or sometimes didn't help.

Pregnancy: Childbirth and Breastfeeding

Finding out about pregnancy, childbirth and breastfeeding was, in general, fairly straightforward. During my first pregnancy I didn't read very widely but found that what I picked up at the classes run by the National Childbirth Trust was most helpful, as was their literature. To find out about classes, their literature and their nursing bras (the best designed I know of), contact their headquarters at 9 Queensborough Terrace, London W2, tel: 01-229 9319. In contrast, I found *Pregnancy Month by Month* (Consumer's Association) of limited informational value and the pamphlets dished out by the ante-natal clinic, whilst better than nothing, of even less use. Although well informed in general, I realised how ignorant I was of anything the slightest bit abnormal when Will arrived prematurely. I wished then that I knew more, for I would have had a store of information to allay some of my bewilderment in those first 24 hours after his birth.

The second time around I made sure that I was considerably better informed. I added to the knowledge I had already acquired in a variety of ways, including reading

Gordon Bourne's *Pregnancy* (Pan Books) which I read from cover to cover and found useful, detailed and informative. Whilst I consumed every bit of information about pregnancy and childbirth, I found myself considerably less concerned about the actual birth than I had been in my first pregnancy. It was not just that I had already had one reasonably easy labour, but that I knew the hospital had an enlightened and progressive attitude towards childbirth. My registering at St. A's the second time was an informed and conscious choice. At that time Sheila Kitzinger's *The Good Birth Guide* (Fontana) had not yet been published, but if it had been I would have been reassured by the fact that her book gave it a star rating.

Having acquired as much information as I could, particularly about what could "go wrong", there was little I could do about controlling the course of events except to take every step I knew to ensure that nothing went wrong. The one exception to that and the one action I did take which could have altered the course of events was to have an amniocentecis. Books on pregnancy, if they mention it at all, only explain what amniocentecis is, how it's done and for what purpose. They do not advise for or against it. Having tried to find out as much about the pros and cons as I could, largely by asking different medical practitioners, and of course taking into account my own case history I finally made my decision on the advice of the doctor in whom I had most confidence.

Funnily enough the area in which I was given the most conflicting advice was breastfeeding. During the long six weeks of struggle to establish breastfeeding with Will, everyone – doctors, nurses, grannies, friends and relatives, all offered different opinions. I supplemented their advice with some reading and found the leaflet published by the National Childbirth Trust the clearest and best on the subject. At the hospital the one person who did give me some factual information about breastfeeding was the paediatric senior registrar although at no time did he tell me that sucking was often a problem for Down's Syndrome babies. Telling me that would not have made the task easier but it would have made me feel less of a failure at certain moments during those six weeks.

Feeding Jessie presented no problems but whilst I was feeding her Ed bought a book called *The Womanly Art of Breastfeeding* (Tandem). There is some useful information and advice in it, but most of it is so taken up with enthusing about breastfeeding as the achievement of full womanliness that we both fluctuated between laughing at it and being appalled by its reactionary attitudes.

Handicap – Mental and Physical

The problem with the information relating to Will's Down's Syndrome was not that the information didn't exist but that it was hard to find. You can't walk into an ordinary bookshop and buy a book on Down's Syndrome as you can on pregnancy. Most people we met were either as ignorant as ourselves or, in the case of the medical personnel we were dealing with, their knowledge was related primarily to physical problems and even then they seemed reluctant to impart that knowledge. It was from acquaintances, mainly through chance remarks either by myself or by friends to friends, that I gained access to information and supportive advice. At least finding out about relevant organisations and self-help groups has been made much easier now by such publications as *Health Help* (available free from HELP, Thames TV, 149 Tottenham Court Rd, London W1).

Some of the first material I read was either pathetically inadequate or depressing or both. A pamphlet called *Your Down's Syndrome Child* by David Pitt M.D. (National Association for Mental Health, Texas, USA) was pathetically inadequate and *Your Mongol Baby* (MIND – National Association for Mental Health) was both inadequate and depressing, neither giving much information nor much hope. MIND have since withdrawn the pamphlet from sale. We did not have any direct contact with MIND during Will's life but since then I have been impressed with the radical approach they adopt to questions of mental health. (MIND – National Association for Mental Health, 22 Harley St, London W1, tel: 01-637 0741).

The first organisation we approached directly was the National Society for Mentally Handicapped Children – NSMHC (National Headquarters and Bookshop – 117 Golden Lane, London EC1, tel: 01-253 9433). We came away from our visit there having gained little. However their bookshop proved to have not only their own publications but also a wider collection of books, pamphlets and other useful information than I have seen elsewhere.

I bought two pamphlets published by them called *The Child with Mongolism* and *Judith: Teaching our Mongol Baby*. Whilst I found neither very informative they were at least positive in approach. I also bought *Parents and Mentally Handicapped Children* by Charles Hannam (Penguin, in association with MIND). Through interviews with parents of mentally handicapped children, the book reveals the difficulties, stresses and strains of being the parent of such a child in a society that offers little support or help. I found it profoundly depressing and managed to read it only with great difficulty, not wishing to contemplate such a future. But the book is useful particularly for the recommendations which it makes for change – changes which if brought about would greatly lessen the burden on parents and improve considerably the life and opportunities of mentally handicapped children.

At a subsequent visit to the bookshop I bought *Improving Babies With Down's Syndrome* by Rex Brinkworth and Dr Joseph Collins (NSMHC). I read it immediately from cover to cover, re-read it and then went back again to certain sections. The book gave me a new lease of life. It not only had more information about Down's Syndrome than I had managed to glean from any other source but it also gave practical guidance as to what one could do to help one's child develop. It was also entirely free of the patronising tone which so many authors, particularly those who are not themselves parents of handicapped children, tend to adopt. Soon I learnt, not to my surprise, that Rex Brinkworth was the founder of the organisation which proved to be of most help to us, the Down's Babies Association now called the Down's Children's Association (Quinborne Community Centre, Ridgacre Rd, Quinton, Birmingham B32 2TW, tel: 021-427 1374).

When I joined the organisation it was very much Birmingham centred with only one or two regional branches. It has now grown and there are regional branches and local groups in most areas. The "Training Schedules" (now called "Parents' Guide") which they send to members are full of information, explanation and practical guidance. Like most other similar organisations they also provided reading lists covering all the literature available on Down's Syndrome and sent out to members a newsletter. The latter I found not only a useful source of additional information but also a source of strength. It was reassuring to belong to an organisation whose other members shared my attitude and shared the desire to improve the future for ourselves and our children.

Anticipating future problems I bought a few leaflets on specific problems, like toilet training a retarded child or speech therapy, but they were left unread. I also bought one or two general books about play designed for parents of normal children. The best by far of these was *Play with a Purpose for Under-Sevens* by E. M. Matterson (Penguin).

Of all the books I read the most exceptional was one lent to me by the mother of a mongol girl. It is the only book written by a Down's Syndrome child and is called *The World of Nigel Hunt* by Nigel Hunt (Darwin Finlayson). It is bizarre, amusing and revealing, particularly of Nigel's enthusiastic approach to life. The portrait he paints of his world is far removed from the dull vacant image too often portrayed of the mentally handicapped child. It was enormously encouraging to read, not only for its content but also for the mere fact of its existence – that a mongol child was literate, in fact more literate than some 'normal' adults.

The other major informational problem we had was finding out about Will's physical difficulties, particularly his heart condition. Although we realised the doctors themselves had had difficulty in diagnosing his heart defect and in putting together a picture of its nature and extent, all too frequently they made little effort to explain to us what they knew in comprehensible language. When a full explanation was given to me by a senior registrar, it showed how, with the aid of a large clear diagram of the heart, its chambers, blood flow system, relationship to lungs, kidneys and so on, doctors *can* explain a serious heart defect in an understandable way and even point out possible areas of complications. The diagram seemed such an obvious visual aid to the doctor that, in retrospect, I cannot understand why all doctors in general practice and in hospitals are not similarly equipped. A variety of problems could then much more clearly and comprehensibly be explained to patients and relatives of patients.

Grief

The area that was most difficult to get advice on was grief. What I did find out was through my own experience and that process of learning continues.

At the time of my greatest need I found no direct help. The general support we had from family and friends, whilst of great importance did not fulfil my particular need for understanding and counselling. Such help could only come, I felt, from someone who had been through a similar experience or possibly from someone who was experienced in talking with people in such situations. Too late for my needs I found out about an organisation called Compassionate Friends who had come into being to offer precisely the kind of understanding, support and advice which I had looked for. Sadly, despite attempts at publicity, their existence is not nearly widely enough known. Although they hope that newly bereaved parents will be referred to them by "nurses, doctors, social workers or anyone who comes into contact with bereaved parents", in my experience no one knew about Compassionate Friends or if they did, they did not see it as their responsibility to refer me to it.

Compassionate Friends describes itself as "An international organisation of bereaved parents offering friendship and understanding to other bereaved parents". It operates by members contacting bereaved parents and, through visits, letters, phone calls and meetings, offering newly bereaved parents both the chance to talk to, and to share their experience with, other bereaved parents. Most importantly they offer long term support, giving members mutual help and understanding when friends and relatives assume that you are over your grief and have returned to emotional normality. The organisation is nationwide, with regional secretaries in most counties. The national secretary, Ms Charmion Mann, can be contacted at 25 Kingsdown Parade, Bristol BS6 5UE, tel: 0272-47316.

For some reason I neither sought, nor did anyone recommend to me, any literature on grief. In the absence of sharing directly the experience reading about someone else's experience can be helpful. The Compassionate Friends have a newsletter which, besides giving information about the organisation, publishes short pieces written by members on their thoughts and feelings about their grief. In addition they have a library for members.

It was also only very recently that quite unexpectedly I read something which made me realise that until then I had not read anything about grief. It made me realise, too, that the reading of something perceptive on the subject could give me greater understanding of my own experience. This book was Vera Brittain's *Testament of Youth* (Fontana). Although the bereavements she suffered were of her contemporaries, not of a child, I found that I not only identified with her descriptions of grief but gained insights into and understanding of some of my own feelings and behaviour.